MARY BURGESS has worked as a Cognitive Behavioral Psychotherapist in the area of chronic fatigue syndrome (CFS) for over ten years. In addition to her clinical work she has been engaged in research and development. This has mainly involved developing and evaluating forms of intervention for patients with CFS, who for whatever reason, have experienced difficulty in getting to the hospital. With colleagues this work has been published in academic journals and has lead to the writing of this book.

A current research interest involves developing a home-based cognitive behavioral program for children who are severely disabled by symptoms of CFS.

TRUDIE CHALDER is Professor of Cognitive Behavioral Psychotherapy at the Institute of Psychiatry at Guy's, King's and St Thomas's School of Medicine (GKT) London. She has worked as a clinician and a researcher in the area of CFS in adults and children for about 17 years. She and colleagues developed the cognitive behavioral treatment of CFS and the approach has now been evaluated in a number of clinical research trials with positive outcomes.

Her more recent research interests include cognitive and behavioral models and treatment of irritable bowel syndrome and diabetes.

The aim of the **Overcoming** series is to enable people with a range of common problems and disorders to take control of their own recovery program. Each title, with its specially tailored program, is devised by a practising clinician using the latest techniques of cognitive behavioral therapy – techniques which have been shown to be highly effective in changing the way people think about themselves and their problems.

The series was initiated in 1993 by Peter Cooper, Professor of Psychology at Reading University and Research Fellow at the University of Cambridge in the UK, whose original volume on overcoming Bulimia Nervosa and Binge-Eating continues to help many people in the USA, the UK, and Europe. Many books in the **Overcoming** series are recommended by the UK Department of Health under the Books on Prescription Scheme.

All titles in the series are available by mail order.
Please see the order form at the back of this book.

OVERCOMING CHRONIC FATIGUE

A self-help guide using
Cognitive Behavioral Techniques

Mary Burgess
with Trudie Chalder

ROBINSON
London

To Marti~~n and my~~ Anna

162 Fulham Palace Road
London W6 9ER
www.constablerobinson.com

First published in the UK by Robinson,
an imprint of Constable & Robinson Ltd 2005

Important Note
This book is not intended to be substitute for medical advice or treatment.
Any person with a condition requiring medical attention should consult a
qualified medical practitioner or suitable therapist.

The information provided on schemes and benefits is only a general guide
and is not a full and authoritative statement of the law. Every effort has
been made to ensure that the information is correct at the date of
publication of this book. However, changes in the law may make the
information become gradually less accurate.

ISBN 1-84119-942-7

Printed and bound in the EU

1 3 5 7 9 10 8 6 4 2

Contents

Contents

Acknowledgements

This book has been developed over the course of many years and a huge number of people have contributed to this final product. We would like first to mention the considerable number of people with chronic fatigue syndrome who have used the techniques described in this book and have made suggestions on how our work could be improved. We would also like to thank all of our colleagues, past and present, who have commented on the text or who have given us feedback from their patients who have used the techniques.

The source of the physiological explanation for chronic fatigue syndrome and some of the information contained within the section on autonomic arousal in CFS came from an unpublished treatment manual written by Pauline Powell, a physiotherapist in Liverpool.

The chapter on overcoming unhelpful thinking patterns was influenced by work carried out by Christine Padesky and Dennis Greenberger; for more comprehensive explanations of the ideas contained within this chapter, we recommend that you refer to their book *Mind over Mood* (for details see Chapter 14, 'Useful Resources').

A personal note from Mary: I would like to thank Trudie Chalder, with whom I have worked for the past ten years. Without her enthusiasm for finding ways to help people with chronic fatigue syndrome, this book might never have been written. Trudie's extensive research and vast clinical experience have contributed not only to our understanding of chronic fatigue syndrome today but also to the development of techniques to help individuals overcome their problems.

Preface

Fatigue is central to many chronic and debilitating illnesses, including chronic fatigue syndrome, chronic pain, cancer, and chronic respiratory problems. However, fatigue is something that also occurs when we are overcommitted, working too hard, or making too little time for relaxation. Although this book has been specifically written for people suffering from chronic fatigue syndrome, many of the techniques will be useful for people who feel fatigued from other causes.

Our reasons for writing a self-help book for people with chronic fatigue syndrome were varied. First, we had carried out a small research study at King's College Hospital, London, which indicated that some patients improved after using an earlier version of this self-help book with only phone calls from a therapist, rather than face-to-face consultations. Second, there are a number of people suffering from chronic fatigue syndrome who do not have access to a clinician with the expertise to help them to overcome their problems. Third, some people suffering from chronic fatigue syndrome continue to lead busy lives that make it difficult for them to attend regular appointments.

The overall aim of this book is to provide you with information and strategies to help you to overcome your fatigue and the restrictions on your life that result from it. The strategies have been shown to be effective in treating a wide range of illnesses, including chronic fatigue syndrome. However, although the help provided here may be enough to help you overcome your fatigue and associated problems, it may not be sufficient for everyone. For those, advice on where to get further help is offered.

How to Use this Book

The information in this book has been laid out in an order that people have generally found useful. We therefore recommend that you work your way through the book in the order that it has been written. When you reach Part Two, the core of the self-help manual, we suggest that you read each chapter more than once before embarking on the suggested strategies. We have suggested a timetable to help you pace your efforts. We also ask you to keep a number of diaries; you may photocopy the blanks provided here for your own use, or alternatively you might prefer to devise your own diary sheets, perhaps on a computer. We suggest that you work through Part Three of the book when you have already made some changes in your life and feel confident with some of the techniques you have learned. If you have relatives or friends who are keen to support you, we suggest you ask them to read Part Four, Chapter 15.

What Does this Book Include?

Part One of this book aims to help you to understand your problem. It describes possible causes of fatigue and discusses factors that may be contributing to maintaining your fatigue. It also gives some possible explanations of other symptoms that are common in people with chronic fatigue syndrome.

Part Two focuses on a variety of practical strategies that aim to help you overcome your fatigue problems. If you feel that not all of the chapters are relevant to your problems, then it is fine to miss out those parts. Before you start applying the various strategies, we would like you to consider 'A Few Words of Warning' on page 33, just to be sure that this approach is right for you.

First of all, you will learn how to monitor your sleep and daytime activities in order to help you decide what you want to change. You will then discover ways of improving the quality of your sleep and regulating your sleep pattern. You will read about how to achieve a better balance between activity and rest, how to set your own targets, and how to work towards them. You will then read a section on how to overcome unhelpful thinking patterns. For people who feel they are not making much progress despite carefully following the instructions in the book, there is a section on how to overcome blocks to recovery. We have also included some strategies on overcoming worry, stress, and anxiety. The final chapter in Part Two discusses practical ways of managing setbacks; you would be advised to read this section with particular care if you notice that your symptoms not only persist but increase substantially.

Part Three focuses on helping you to consolidate what you have learned, and prepares you for maintaining and making further progress. It begins with a section of case studies that will help you see how other people have tackled similar problems to those you may be facing. Information on where to get further help and a reading list are also provided.

Finally, Part Four offers some brief guidelines and information for your partner, relatives, and close friends. The aim of this chapter is to help the people close to you to understand your fatigue problems and to offer you support as and when you need it.

PART ONE

Understanding Chronic Fatigue Syndrome

1

What Is Chronic Fatigue Syndrome?

In this chapter we give you some background information about chronic fatigue syndrome and discuss factors that may contribute to its onset. We also offer some explanations for many of the common symptoms experienced by people with chronic fatigue syndrome and discuss some of the treatments that are available.

What Is Fatigue?

Fatigue is a difficult concept as it means different things to different people. People will often describe their fatigue using words such as *weakness, profound tiredness* or *sleepiness*, a *complete lack of energy* or *feeling totally drained*. Fatigue feels very different from the normal sort of tiredness experienced by a healthy person and is often associated with other feelings, such as pain, irritability, frustration, and sometimes low mood or anxiety. Fatigue is often a signal to stop or reduce activity, although paradoxically there is evidence that inactivity produces chronic fatigue; we will return to this topic later in the book.

Fatigue is a very common problem, affecting up to 30 per cent of the UK population (20 per cent of the US population) at any one time. It is a symptom that can be associated with many illnesses. However, a single explanation for fatigue is rarely found. Fatigue often develops following an infection, and sometimes

3

occurs when life is very busy and stressful. Whatever the cause of your fatigue, it is a *real* and debilitating problem.

What Is Chronic Fatigue Syndrome?

Chronic fatigue syndrome (CFS), also known as post-viral fatigue syndrome (PVFS) or myalgic encephalomyelitis (ME), is an illness that has attracted much attention over recent years. Agreeing a name for the illness has been problematic as there has been much debate about the relative contributions of 'physiological' and 'psychological' factors in its development. This outmoded, dualistic view of illness assumes that the body and mind work separately and is unhelpful in understanding any condition. We will be offering alternative ways of viewing CFS later on.

Chronic fatigue syndrome is a fairly new label, although the illness itself was clearly described more than a hundred years ago. At that time it was called *neurasthenia*.

The main symptom experienced by people with CFS is persistent fatigue which feels overwhelming and unlike normal tiredness. Other symptoms may include painful muscles and/or joints, sore throat, headaches, pins and needles, dizziness, and sensitivity to light and noise. CFS has some marked similarities to fibromyalgia, a disorder involving widespread musculoskeletal pain and fatigue; however, the component of muscle pain in fibromyalgia is generally higher. People with CFS often report impairments of their thinking, such as poor concentration, difficulty in finding words, and impaired short-term memory. Problems with sleep are also common; for example, difficulty getting to sleep, sleeping for very long periods, restless sleep with frequent dreams, waking frequently, sleeping but waking unrefreshed. Many people with CFS also report digestive disturbances such as bloating, nausea, or loss of appetite. Food intolerances and increased sensitivity to some foods, alcohol, and substances containing caffeine, such as tea and coffee, are often reported.

Symptoms vary among individuals and may come and go. However, whatever combination they take, they are usually very debilitating and lead many sufferers to make radical changes to their lifestyles. For some people this means giving up work or studying; alternatively, or in addition, it may mean reducing or restricting social and leisure activities and what they can do at home or with their family. The severity of the symptoms may leave people feeling so exhausted that they remain in bed for most of the day. Others may be able to go to work or manage their home, but do little else. Most find that their symptoms are made worse by physical and mental exertion. As a result of this disabling illness, people with CFS will sometimes complain of feelings of frustration, helplessness, and low mood.

How Is Chronic Fatigue Syndrome Diagnosed?

As with many other illnesses where there is no known single cause, for example irritable bowel syndrome (IBS), there is no test to diagnose chronic fatigue syndrome. A diagnosis of CFS is usually made by taking a detailed account of the symptoms, including how they started, how they behave (e.g. whether they worsen in response to certain activities), and the length of time they have been occurring. Basic screening blood tests will also be carried out to rule out any other illnesses that may account for the symptoms. Other more specialist tests are sometimes conducted, for example if there is significant weight loss or a history of foreign travel, but this depends on the symptoms. Medical practitioners can make the diagnosis of CFS, but sometimes they prefer to refer patients to a specialist with an interest in CFS.

How Common Is Chronic Fatigue Syndrome?

It is difficult to say precisely how common chronic fatigue syndrome is in the general population. First, it depends on how chronic fatigue syndrome is defined. Second, although some people may have all the symptoms of CFS, they may not attribute them to the illness itself.

Although 10–30 per cent of all UK patients going to see their doctor for any reason report substantial fatigue lasting for more than a few weeks (15–27 per cent in the US), studies have indicated that a diagnosis of chronic fatigue syndrome is made in only a small minority of these cases. CFS appears to be more common in women than men. A variety of explanations have been put forward for this, in particular changes in the role of women, with increased demands and expectations. Although fatigue is relatively uncommon during childhood, its incidence rises during adolescence. Chronic fatigue syndrome can occur at any time in adulthood.

What Causes Chronic Fatigue Syndrome?

As we noted above, it appears that there is no single cause of CFS. People report a variety of different things that happened at the beginning of their illness, including different types of illness or infection; but some were not aware of any infection or illness at all. Some sufferers can pinpoint the exact date that their CFS started; for others, the onset is more gradual. In the face of this wide range of experience, it is unlikely that a single cause for CFS will ever be identified. However, there is a growing body of evidence that suggests that a number of factors may be involved in triggering the illness.

If you have chronic fatigue syndrome, it is likely that you will be able to identify with some, though probably not all, of the triggers listed below.

Infection

The starting point of CFS is often identified with an initial illness, frequently in the form of a viral infection: for example, a cold, influenza, or glandular fever. Serious viral infections can make us feel tired for up to six months.

Sometimes people report having had a series of infections, which may be a sign that they are run down. However, there is no clear evidence of the virus or bacterium persisting once CFS has become established. Recent research suggests that excessive resting at the height of an infection is likely to lead to worse symptoms several weeks and months later. Although it is pertinent to 'take it easy' when in the acute phase of an infection, too much rest is unhelpful.

Lifestyle

Fatigue can develop in association with a busy lifestyle. Leading a life which allows little time for relaxation is stressful. Following an infection or other illness, a person may feel under pressure to meet their previous levels of commitment, whether at work or at home, and this may lead to exhaustion. Being too busy is as likely to lead to fatigue as being inactive.

Life Events

Changing jobs, getting married, pregnancy, moving house, a bereavement, ending a long-term relationship: all these are stressful events which may lead to increased vulnerability to CFS.

Personality

People with CFS often report that they are hardworking and conscientious, and have high expectations of themselves. Individuals with this type of personality tend to strive very hard to achieve in all they do, leaving little time for pleasure or relaxation. This then feeds into the 'lifestyle' trigger identified above.

Not everyone, however, will recognize these contributory causes. Some people will report that their condition developed for no apparent reason, simply coming out of the blue.

What Keeps the Chronic Fatigue Problem Going?

Just as there are many factors involved in triggering CFS, there are also many factors that are involved in keeping it going. These include the following.

Resuming Normal Activities Too Soon after an Initial Infection

If you keep up your usual level of activity – whether work, exercise, or child care – when you have an infection, or resume that level almost immediately, then your recovery is likely to take longer.

Resting Too Much

Although resting for a short time is the correct thing to do when you have an acute illness or infection, prolonged rest can impede recovery and cause its own set of problems. Evidence clearly suggests that the longer you rest when you have a viral illness, the more symptoms you will have six months later. Prolonged rest makes it harder to become active again and actually increases fatigue. Resting for too long will affect the cardiovascular system, nervous system and musculoskeletal system. Further details of the physical effects of CFS are given in the next section of this chapter, entitled 'Physiological Aspects of Chronic Fatigue Syndrome'.

Receiving Confusing Messages about the Illness Itself and How to Deal with It

Many people with CFS will have sought advice or treatment from a number of sources, received a variety of different messages, and tried a range of different treatments. Many people report being told by well-meaning health professionals that they should rest at the onset and are frequently encouraged to rest for too long. This advice is often accompanied by fear-inducing messages that not resting will lead to prolonged illness. This can all too easily leave the sufferer feeling baffled about what to do for the best and further wearied by the effort of trying to find a potential 'cure'.

Overvigorous Activity Alternating with Resting for Long Periods

Some people refer to this as a 'boom and bust pattern': that is, doing too much when you have some energy, with the result that you then feel even more fatigued and have to rest for longer afterwards. This pattern of activity exacerbates the problem in the longer term, as it makes it difficult to establish any type of routine.

Disturbed Sleep Pattern

Going to bed and getting up at irregular times, or resting too much in the day, may contribute to disturbed and unrefreshing sleep at night. Not sleeping well at night is likely to increase feelings of fatigue and other symptoms of CFS.

Focusing on Symptoms

The symptoms commonly experienced by people with CFS are both distressing and debilitating, and it is therefore understandable that from time to time you may worry about them. Unfortunately, symptoms thrive on attention: in other words, the more you focus on your symptoms, the worse they are likely to get.

Worries about Activity Making the Illness Worse

People with CFS commonly experience increased pain or fatigue after *any* activity, and many understandably read this as a sign that they are doing harm to their bodies. If you have worries like these, you may have reduced your activities and rested for long periods in the belief that resting will help you to feel better. However, as we have already mentioned, resting for too long can cause its own set of problems.

Life Stress and Low Mood

Many people with CFS experience significant and continuing stresses and problems in their lives as a result of their illness. These may include one or more of the following:

- financial difficulties arising from having given up work or reduced working hours;
- worries about holding down a job or keeping up with studies;
- anxiety about a changed role within the family through being less able to take responsibility for dependants;
- reduced social contacts, leading to feelings of isolation;
- feelings of guilt about not being a 'good' parent/wife/husband, etc.

These stresses and anxieties can understandably trigger feelings such as frustration, helplessness, and a sense of loss of control over life. These feelings in turn can lead to low mood, and even to depression. Low mood can lead to a variety of problems, including tiredness, which can further reduce the desire to be active.

Physiological Aspects of Chronic Fatigue Syndrome

Many people with CFS are concerned that their distressing symptoms may be related to a disease that hasn't been detected. Others, who had a viral infection at the time their CFS began, are concerned that the virus is still present or has caused damage to the body. Intensive research has tried to establish a physiological explanation for the very distressing and debilitating symptoms experienced by people with CFS.

Over time, reduced or irregular activity and increased periods of rest cause physical changes in the body. These changes can both exacerbate the unpleasant sensations of CFS and cause additional symptoms such as increased muscle pain on exercise. It is important to point out that these changes are reversible with physical rehabilitation and/or exercise.

Researchers have looked at the effects of rest in healthy people when they reduce their activities, and many similarities between healthy inactive people and people with CFS have been noted. The following paragraphs describe the effects on the body of prolonged periods of inactivity, and how these effects are experienced.

Changes in Muscle Function

A decrease in the number of active cell mitochondria (tiny parts of the cell that produce energy) and their enzymes has been found in the muscles of CFS patients when compared with healthy *active* people. This reduction of cell mitochondria has also been found in healthy *inactive* people. Fewer cell mitochondria may lead to production of lactic acid at low exercise levels, which in turn limits muscle performance.

These changes may account for the feeling of a lack of power or energy in the muscles.

Reduced activity leads to muscles being less efficient (reduced in strength, tone, and size), and consequently less effective in squeezing the blood back to the heart; this causes blood to pool in the lower part of the legs.

Pooling of blood can cause pain both during activity and at rest.

When muscles are not used regularly, they become unfit or deconditioned. When these muscles contract during activity, uneven stresses are produced.

This may result in a feeling of weakness and unsteadiness followed by delayed pain and discomfort.

In respect of this last point, it is important to note that for everyone muscle pain and stiffness are natural consequences of beginning a new exercise program or taking exercise to which they are unaccustomed. They are therefore not an indication that the exercise should be halted; only that it should be built up gradually.

11

Changes in the Cardiovascular System

The cardiovascular system (which incorporates the heart and blood vessels) loses condition very quickly with rest. The longer you rest, the more changes occur.

Physical changes that occur with cardiovascular deconditioning include:

- after one or two days' bed rest, reduced blood volume; after eight days' bed rest, reduced volume of red blood cells, which reduces the oxygen-carrying capacity of the blood;
- after 20 days' bed rest, the volume of the heart reduces by about 15 per cent, so that less blood is pumped to other organs.

The physical changes described above may result in making you feel breathless or dizzy when exercising, and contribute to your fatigue.

Following a 'lying down' rest there is a drop in blood pressure on standing up (postural hypotension) as gravity causes blood to pool in the limbs. Consequently, less blood returns to the heart and therefore less blood goes to the brain. Restricting salt or liquid intake reduces blood volume and can exacerbate dizziness on standing up.

The reduced blood flow to the brain causes dizziness and sometimes fainting on standing up.

Regulation of Body Temperature

Changes in the blood flow to major body organs occur following prolonged rest, and these lead to changes in surface body temperature.

This may result in feeling hot and/or cold, with excessive and inappropriate sweating at times.

Changes in Sight and Hearing

Prolonged bed rest results in a 'headward' shift of bodily fluids.
This may result in visual problems and sensitivity to noise.

Reduced Tolerance to Activity or Exercise

General deconditioning of the body occurs as a result of prolonged rest or reduced activity.

As fitness reduces, it is harder work to be active. Muscle fatigue and feelings of heaviness, as well as a general increase in overall fatigue, occur when activity is resumed.

During periods of prolonged physical or mental exertion, the nervous system is more active than normal and adrenaline production is raised. This leads to symptoms similar to those experienced in a flu-like illness, such as *aches and pains, headache, sweating, feeling hot and cold, chest tightness,* and *sore throat.* If a person experiences these symptoms after activity, they may reduce or avoid activities, as they may believe that they are coming down with flu or a cold. Limiting activity can perpetuate the symptoms and lead to a further reduction of fitness and muscle strength.

Changes in the Nervous System

One of the functions of the nervous system is to coordinate the muscles. Regular performance of an activity is required to maintain good coordination. Prolonged periods of inactivity therefore reduce coordination.

This may result in unsteadiness, clumsiness, and reduced accuracy on carrying out precise movements.

Changes in Mental Functioning

Prolonged rest deprives people of intellectual stimulation and has a dulling effect on intellectual activity.

This may impair concentration, memory, and the ability to find the correct word.

Alteration of the Biological Clock

The 'biological clock', which is located in a part of the brain called the hypothalamus, regulates many body rhythms that run on an approximate 24-hour cycle. These rhythms are called 'circadian rhythms', and they control vital functions such as:

- sleeping and waking;
- feelings of tiredness and alertness;
- intellectual performance;
- memory;
- appetite;
- body temperature;
- the production of hormones; e.g. cortisol (which is important in regulating our metabolism);
- the activity of the immune system.

Circadian rhythms are responsible for the body 'feeling' things at certain times of the day: for example, hunger, alertness, tiredness, the need to go to the bathroom. The biological clock is affected by the events of the day and is reset each day by cues such as times of getting up or going to bed, mealtimes, and performing daily routines. If these cues do not occur, the biological clock's timekeeping can be disturbed; this can happen, for example, when flying across different time-zones (jet-lag), working shifts – or experiencing illness.

If regular cues are lost, disruption of the clock results in a slipping of body rhythms that can lead to:

- the 'normal' intense feelings of tiredness at night shifting into the day, making it difficult to cope with your usual daytime routine;
- the 'normal' daytime rhythm shifting to the night, making you more alert and causing difficulty in getting to sleep.

This in turn can lead to:

- poor-quality sleep at night;
- increasing fatigue during the day;
- poor concentration and forgetfulness;
- low mood;
- feeling generally unwell;

- headaches;
- muscle aches;
- loss of appetite;
- irregularities of bowel movement.

As the symptoms of chronic fatigue syndrome are similar to those of jet-lag, circadian rhythms of people with CFS have been investigated. Evidence from some studies indicates that CFS is associated with the biological clock losing control of the body rhythms.

What may happen is an infection, a very stressful life event, or an accumulation of persistent stress causes worry and disturbs sleep at night. This leads to irregular times of getting up and going to bed, and more rests taken during the day. Thus the usual daily routine and normal sleep–waking cycle, both needed to reset the biological clock, are disrupted. The biological clock then loses control over body rhythms, resulting in the mental and physical symptoms of CFS.

Disturbance of Cortisol Production

Cortisol is a hormone whose production is controlled by a circadian rhythm. It sets our metabolism in action in the morning to prepare us for the physical and mental challenges of the day. Exercise, other activity, and stress cause an increase in the level of cortisol in the bloodstream.

Low cortisol levels have been found in people who have disrupted sleep, such as healthy individuals who have rested in bed for more than three weeks, healthy workers after working five night shifts, and people suffering from jet-lag.

Research shows that some people with CFS also have a lower than normal level of cortisol; it is thought that these low cortisol levels are probably caused by disrupted sleep and irregular activity.

Low cortisol may add to the feeling of tiredness, decreased alertness, and poor performance seen both in people with CFS and those who work on night shifts.

Disturbance of the Sleep–Wake Rhythm

Most people with CFS complain of poor-quality sleep. Common problems include difficulty in getting to sleep, restlessness, waking in the night, and waking feeling unrefreshed and sleepy.

In a study where the sleep patterns of healthy volunteers were deliberately disrupted to make them similar to those of people with CFS, they developed symptoms similar to those of CFS, including feeling unrefreshed and physically weak, sleepiness, poor concentration, and muscle aches. However, when they were allowed to sleep undisturbed, their symptoms subsided. This study indicates that a disturbed sleep pattern can cause some symptoms of CFS, but that these symptoms are reversible.

Disruption of sleep can affect the activity of the immune system, possibly increasing vulnerability to colds and infection. *Inactivity and being deprived of sleep cause an increase in the feelings of effort and fatigue when performing activity or exercise.*

Autonomic Arousal in Chronic Fatigue Syndrome

Autonomic arousal is an automatic physical response of the body to a threatening or stressful situation. We can all remember having butterflies before an exam, an interview, or going to the dentist! When we are in a situation that makes us feel anxious, the central nervous system becomes more active and an increased amount of the hormone adrenaline is released into the bloodstream. These natural changes have a protective function in preparing us for action to counter a threatened danger; however, the physical feelings that we experience when anxious can be very unpleasant.

Having CFS can at times be very stressful. You may be not only dealing with your illness, but also facing other concerns related to it, such as financial worries and/or an inability to meet deadlines at work, college, or home. You may worry about whether you are making your symptoms worse by following advice that you have been given. You also may worry about the causes of your condition and the effects of CFS on your own and others' lives. If you have been ill for a while, you may worry about doing things that you haven't done for a long time, such as meeting friends. All of these worries may at times trigger feelings of anxiety, which in turn can lead to a range of unpleasant physical feelings. These effects, and how you may experience them, are listed below.

Increased Heart Rate

This can be felt as a racing pulse, palpitations, pounding, or tightness in the chest.

Some people feel very frightened by these sensations and so become yet more anxious, resulting in a further release of adrenaline that maintains the physical sensations.

Increase in Blood Pressure

High blood pressure is noted in some people with anxiety. This is likely to be associated with an exaggerated autonomic response to stress by the nervous system.

There are usually no particular signs or symptoms of high blood pressure; it is usually detected only in the course of routine investigations by doctors or if another illness is present; for example, heart or kidney problems.

Breathlessness, Which Can Lead to Hyperventilation

This natural response to being anxious enables our lungs to be filled with oxygen to prepare us for action. However, if over-breathing (hyperventilation) continues for a while, an array of unpleasant symptoms may occur because it reduces the amount of carbon dioxide in the blood. This changes the balance of chemicals in the blood, causing tightening of the blood vessels and reduced blood supply, especially in the brain.

This reduced blood supply to the brain causes sensations such as light-headedness, dizziness, feeling faint, feeling unsteady, blurred vision, pins and needles, tingling, or numbness (sometimes one-sided) in the limbs or face, or clumsiness. Cramplike muscle spasms may be experienced, particularly in the hands and feet. Increased sensitivity to light and noise may also occur, as well as abnormal sensations such as feelings of being detached from oneself. Feelings of unreality or being out of control may also occur.

Feelings of faintness are misleading, because blood pressure is usually high in anxiety and fainting occurs only when blood pressure is very low. However, anxiety may precede a faint when someone who has a blood and injury phobia has an injection or sees blood: in these situations blood pressure drops and fainting can occur.

The muscles of the chest wall can be overused during hyperventilation, which may lead to *chest pain* or *discomfort*. If these sensations are interpreted as signs of a serious problem, for example of heart trouble, that can lead to a further increase in anxiety and adrenaline production, leading to a further increase of unpleasant sensations.

Overbreathing also results in increased use of the muscles of the head, neck, and shoulders, resulting in headaches and localized stiffness and pain.

Overuse of the neck muscles in hyperventilation can be accompanied by sensations of tightness or soreness in the throat.

Increased nerve activity and release of adrenaline may also cause excessive breathing through the mouth and reduced saliva production. These result in a dry mouth, swallowing difficulties, and the feeling of a lump in the throat.

Altered Blood Flow

When we are anxious, blood is redirected to muscles to prepare for action. Reduced blood flow to the skin may cause *pallor, pain, coldness of hands and feet*, and sometimes *numbness or tingling*.

Reduced blood flow to the bowel affects the passage of food and can result in *symptoms of irritable bowel; for example, constipation and/or diarrhoea and abdominal discomfort.*

Muscle Tension

There is an increase in the tension of the muscles to prepare them for action.

This can cause aches, pains (particularly in the shoulders, neck, jaw, and head), and fatigue. Muscular twitching or trembling may also occur.

Visual Disturbance

Increased nerve activity affects the muscles of the iris (the coloured part of eye), causing the pupils to dilate and so to let in more light. This may help to explain the sensitivity to bright light experienced by some people with CFS. The shape of the eye lens is altered to help improve side and distance vision. Together, the effects of these changes can be experienced as *blurring of vision.*

Sweating

Increased sweating occurs to allow for heat loss, causing *clammy hands and feet.*

Sleep Disturbance

Adrenaline production increases at times of stress, so that sleep disturbance, for example *difficulty getting to sleep* or *frequent waking,* is very common; it may be accompanied by *nightmares* and *sweating.*

Mental Functioning

Anxiety may affect mental functioning in a number of ways and contribute to the following:

- mood disturbance; for example, irritability, being easily upset;
- inability to concentrate, forgetfulness, indecisiveness;

restlessness; for example, being fidgety or unable to sit still;
- a tendency to go over things again and again.

Everyone experiences physical symptoms of anxiety in an individual way, and few people have all of the symptoms listed above. However, when any of these symptoms are extreme, they can easily be misinterpreted as signs of a serious disease, and worry about this can trigger further unpleasant symptoms; this vicious circle can occasionally trigger a panic attack.

An increase in nerve activity and adrenaline production can precipitate feelings of weakness and exhaustion on top of the fatigue and muscle aches of chronic fatigue syndrome.

Management of Chronic Fatigue Syndrome

Every person who has chronic fatigue syndrome has a different story to tell about what they have been advised to do by health professionals. This account will vary according to the beliefs or knowledge about CFS of the health-care professionals that you see; the availability of specialists in this area of medicine; and access to information about CFS: for example, through local support groups, the Internet, and so on.

You may feel that your illness has not been taken seriously. You may have been told that there is nothing wrong with you, that it is all in your mind, or that you should pull yourself together. On the other hand, you may have been told to rest until you feel better – or, conversely, to do as much as you can. You may have tried a number of remedies; or you may be reading this book without ever having talked to anyone about your chronic fatigue.

Even if a physical cause of your symptoms cannot be found, that does not mean there is nothing wrong with you. A combination of many factors may have precipitated and be maintaining your CFS. Every illness from the common cold to cancer can be affected by our lifestyle, attitudes, experiences, and other things that happen around us. For example, you may have noticed that you are more likely to have a cold when you are particularly busy and under pressure.

In Part Two of this book we describe practical strategies to help you overcome your CFS. Some of the other treatments and remedies that are commonly used to treat chronic fatigue syndrome are listed here.

Antidepressants

There is little evidence that antidepressants will reduce fatigue in people with chronic fatigue syndrome. However, they may be useful in treating any associated depression. Some antidepressants also contain properties that can alleviate muscle pain and insomnia.

Corticosteroids

There is not enough evidence of the effects of corticosteroids in people with CFS to arrive at any conclusion about their usefulness. Any benefit from low doses has been short-lived, and higher doses have been linked with adverse effects such as adrenal suppression.

Immunotherapy

Again, there is a lack of substantial evidence to support the use of immunotherapy in people with CFS. Adverse effects including headaches, fatigue, and gastrointestinal disturbances have been reported.

Dietary Supplements

Little research has been carried out in this area. One study has shown benefits in some patients having magnesium injections. There have been mixed results from using evening primrose oil.

Diet

Various diets have been recommended in the treatment of chronic fatigue syndrome. If there is a proven allergy or intolerance, there may be benefits in excluding the aggravating food substance. Many people with CFS report being intolerant to alcohol and therefore exclude it from their diet. However, it is worth bearing in mind that avoiding any food for a while will result in a change in gastrointestinal functioning when reintroduced. Alterations in diet when travelling abroad, for example, may have similar effects.

Prolonged Rest

Prolonged rest has not been shown to be helpful in the treatment of CFS. There is a lot of indirect evidence to suggest that prolonged rest may delay recovery because of the associated physical deconditioning.

Graded Exercise

Graded exercise is designed to reverse the physical deconditioning (reduced fitness) and reduced muscle strength found in people who have chronic fatigue syndrome. It has been shown in research trials to reduce fatigue and substantially improve physical functioning for people with CFS.

Pacing

Pacing is an energy management strategy in which people with chronic fatigue syndrome are encouraged to achieve an appropriate balance between rest and activity. This usually involves living within the physical and mental limitations imposed by the illness and avoiding activities that exacerbate symptoms or interspersing activities with planned rests. Pacing has been reported as useful by the UK patient organization Action For ME (AFME), which collated responses from CFS sufferers. Pacing has yet to be evaluated in a randomized research trial.

Complementary and Alternative Medicine

The terms 'complementary' and 'alternative' medicine refer to a wide range of approaches that aim to improve health and well-being. Although they are not generally considered to be part of mainstream medical care, they have been found helpful by people with a wide range of health problems and illnesses, including chronic fatigue syndrome. Although approaches including homoeopathy, osteopathy, acupuncture, and herbal remedies have helped some people with CFS, there is no research evidence to support their use.

2

Understanding Your Own Chronic Fatigue Problems

In the previous chapter we discussed factors that commonly contribute to the onset and maintenance of chronic fatigue syndrome. However, your own particular experience is unique to you, and may include different factors as well as some combination of those we have described. It is worth spending a bit of time at this point considering your own fatigue problems so that you can more easily pinpoint what you will particularly need to focus on.

The Vicious Circle of Fatigue

We often refer to factors that maintain a condition such as fatigue as 'a vicious circle', because one factor leads to another that then reinforces the effect of the first, and so on. Figure 2.1 illustrates how this pattern works, summarizing factors that contribute to the development of chronic fatigue syndrome and illustrating how other factors may contribute to maintaining it. Although it is unlikely that it will completely fit your experience, you may be able to identify with some of it.

In order to help you to understand your chronic fatigue problem better, you may like to use the blank page on page 26 to draw your own vicious circle.

CONTRIBUTING FACTORS

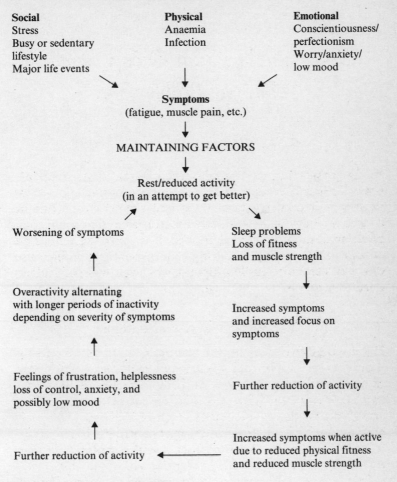

Social
Stress
Busy or sedentary
lifestyle
Major life events

Physical
Anaemia
Infection

Emotional
Conscientiousness/
perfectionism
Worry/anxiety/
low mood

Symptoms
(fatigue, muscle pain, etc.)

MAINTAINING FACTORS

Rest/reduced activity
(in an attempt to get better)

Worsening of symptoms

Sleep problems
Loss of fitness
and muscle strength

Overactivity alternating
with longer periods of inactivity
depending on severity of symptoms

Increased symptoms
and increased focus on
symptoms

Feelings of frustration, helplessness
loss of control, anxiety, and
possibly low mood

Further reduction of activity

Further reduction of activity

Increased symptoms when active
due to reduced physical fitness
and reduced muscle strength

Figure 2.1   A vicious circle of fatigue

My Vicious Circle of Fatigue

PART TWO

Learning How to Cope

Introduction

In this part of the book we aim to help you to tackle some of the things that may have been contributing to keeping your chronic fatigue syndrome going. We hope that, as you follow the strategies outlined here, your symptoms will become less intense or even go away; and that, if some of them do not, you will feel more able to cope with them, so that you will be able to do more of what you would like to do.

The first three chapters in this part set out the framework for the practical work that follows. These will give you a solid foundation on which to base your efforts, and we do recommend that you read through them two or three times before embarking on the following sections.

First, in Chapter 3, we talk about cognitive behavior therapy (CBT) as a treatment for chronic fatigue syndrome. It is important that you know that the techniques included in this book have been used effectively to help people with CFS in research studies, as well as by a variety of specially trained health professionals. We then outline what is involved in applying CBT techniques in a self-help program designed to help overcome CFS. In Chapter 4 we show you how you can gather and record information about your own condition and how you actually live at the moment; for example, when and how you rest and sleep, how much activity you take and when. In Chapter 5 we show how you can set realistic and appropriate targets for yourself. These chapters will enable you to know exactly what you are aiming to achieve and to measure your progress step-by-step. We then move on in Chapters 6–11 to describe the various techniques that will help you to change or adapt the way in which you manage your illness.

3

Cognitive Behavior Therapy for Chronic Fatigue Syndrome

In this chapter, after outlining a few facts about cognitive behavior therapy and how it has been used to treat chronic fatigue syndrome, we discuss what you will be doing to help yourself to overcome your chronic fatigue problems in the next few months. We would like you to pay particular attention to the short section on page 33 entitled 'A Few Words of Warning', as it will help you to clarify whether this is the right approach for you and whether you need to see your doctor before you make a start.

What Is Cognitive Behavior Therapy?

Cognitive behavior therapy (CBT) is a treatment that has been found to be valuable and effective in helping people with many illnesses and disorders, including chronic pain, irritable bowel syndrome, and diabetes, as well as depression, eating disorders, and conditions related to anxiety. CBT focuses on identifying and changing not only patterns of behavior but also the patterns of thought that keep them going – hence the 'cognitive' element alongside the 'behavioral' element in the name.

In the course of their work with various illnesses and conditions, cognitive behavior therapists became aware that many people who could benefit from the approach do not have access to qualified therapists in their area, and that the efforts individuals make to overcome their own problems often actually have the reverse effect, keeping those problems going and sometimes even making them worse. With this in mind, self-help programmes have been developed using the methods and techniques applied in CBT, and these have been found to help many people reduce or eliminate the symptoms of various disorders without recourse to individual therapy (see the front of this book for a list of the disorders tackled by the Overcoming series.). This book offers such a program, aimed at helping individuals to overcome their symptoms of chronic fatigue by following strategies that we have designed according to the principles of CBT and used in our professional therapy practice.

Although many people have been helped to overcome many different illnesses and disorders by using these self-help programs, there are some people for whom they are not appropriate; so again, we urge you to read and consider the section 'A Few Words of Warning' before you embark on the work set out in the following chapters.

Has Any Research Shown that CBT Is Helpful in CFS?

The effectiveness of CBT in treating CFS has been evaluated in three well-conducted research studies undertaken since the 1990s. All three were conducted as randomized controlled trials; that is, trials in which there are more than one treatment group, and participating patients do not know which group they are in. CBT was found to produce better results than the other treatments with which they were compared.

Two of the trials were carried out in the UK. The first, conducted in Oxford, compared CBT with seeing a doctor for 'usual' medical care. At the end of the one-year follow-up period, two-thirds of the participants who had had CBT were functioning at satisfactory levels, compared with only a quarter of those who had been given 'usual' medical care. The second trial, carried out at King's College Hospital, London, compared 13 sessions of CBT with a similar number of sessions of relaxation therapy. Here, too, at the six-month follow-up stage, about two-thirds of patients who had been given CBT achieved satisfactory levels of functioning, compared with about a quarter of those who had received relaxation therapy. At the five-year follow-up point, many of those who had improved through CBT had sustained that improvement.

A third study, carried out in the Netherlands, divided participants into three groups, one receiving CBT, one taking part in a support group, and one receiving no treatment. At the eight-month follow-up, CBT was found to be significantly more effective than either of the 'control' options: approximately half of the patients who had received CBT had improved to a satisfactory level of functioning. There was no difference in outcome between the two control groups.

What Will I Have to Do?

Chapters 4–11 will guide you through the procedures necessary to help you to deal with the various problems associated with your chronic fatigue syndrome. This section summarizes the components of the program.

Monitor Your Activity Levels

To help you to build up an accurate picture of what you are doing each day, you will be asked to complete activity diaries every day for at least a few weeks. These diaries will help you to see at a glance whether there are times when you are doing too little or too much.

Monitor Your Sleep Pattern

To help you to build up an accurate picture of your sleep, you will be asked to complete a sleep diary for a few weeks. This will help you to see at a glance whether or how often you have difficulties with your sleep; for example, taking a long time to go to sleep, waking frequently in the night, sleeping for many hours on some nights and only a few on others, etc.

Set Your Own Targets

Setting targets will help you to focus on what *you* would like to work towards during the next few months. It is a good idea to have targets across a range of areas of life – including, for example, leisure interests and pursuits as well as work and home tasks – so that you are aiming to construct a balanced lifestyle.

Use a Variety of Strategies to Improve Your Sleep

The strategies that you use to improve your sleep will depend on your particular sleep problem(s). For example, if you have no set times for going to bed or waking up, you may find it helpful to learn how to establish a routine. If you have problems going to sleep at night, you will learn strategies to help you to get to sleep more quickly: these may involve developing a routine before going to bed, reducing sleep in the day, and learning to cope with worries that may be keeping you awake.

Stabilize Your Activity and Rests

This will involve planning a program of scheduled activity and rest, which you will review and change every couple of weeks or so. The aim is to carry out the same amount of activity and rest each day, avoiding bursts of activity when feeling well and long periods of rest when fatigued. Introducing short periods of relaxation will be important if you generally do too much.

Increase or Change Your Activities

When you have established a routine, you will be in a position to take steps to work towards your targets. This will involve your gradually increasing some activities (e.g. walking) and introducing new activities (e.g. doing a course); and for some people it may mean *reducing* activities (e.g. ceasing to work very long hours).

Learn How to Overcome Unhelpful Thoughts and Beliefs

This will initially involve identifying thoughts that may be hampering your progress or leaving you feeling frustrated, such as 'I'll never get better' or 'I haven't achieved anything today'. You will learn to challenge these thoughts by coming up with more helpful alternatives.

Learn How to Manage a Setback

Overcoming an illness is hardly ever straightforward. There may be times when your symptoms suddenly increase and you find it more difficult to manage your everyday activities. You will learn how to recognize these difficult times and how to implement strategies to overcome your setback and move forward.

What Can I Expect from Working through This Section?

- You will become more in control of your illness by recognizing your limitations and developing a better balance between activity (e.g. work, chores, socializing) and rest/relaxation.
- You will become competent in reviewing and updating your activity program so that you can gradually work towards your targets.
- You will recognize and deal with any blocks that may be making it difficult for you to progress.
- You will learn how worry and stress may affect you and how to deal with them.
- You will learn how to recognize and manage a setback (an increase in your symptoms).

A Few Words of Warning!

We would expect that most people who read this book will already have seen their doctor to discuss their health problems. If not, we strongly recommend that you do so before you start working through the self-help program. Your doctor will want to take a history of your symptoms and in some cases may want to do a few simple blood tests and maybe a urine test to rule out other diagnoses that may explain your symptoms.

To get the most out of this book, you need to feel able to commit yourself to following its guidelines for some time – generally a period of a few months. This is because a lot of the strategies in this book can take some time to master, and it can take a corresponding length of time to start experiencing the benefits.

Because of the commitment required, it will be important that you choose a good time to start working through the program. Some people may be able to start straight away. However, if, for example, you are in the middle of exams or moving house, or your children are off school for the holidays, it may be best to wait for a calmer period of your life. It can be helpful to view CBT as a course into which you have to put something in order to get something out of it.

It can be helpful to involve a partner, relative, or close friend in your CBT program as a companion, because at times you may find it quite hard to stick to the guidelines. The support of someone close to you may encourage you to keep going. Chapter 15 on pages 197–200 contains some guidelines that will help them to help you.

You are likely to get more out of this program if you do not try anything else new to help your fatigue at the same time. Starting more than one thing at a time can be confusing because when things begin to improve you will not know what is helping.

What Is Likely to Happen to My Symptoms?

The severity and range of symptoms, and their effects on people's lives, vary greatly in people with chronic fatigue syndrome. For some people, their activities have greatly reduced, while others are generally doing too much. A third group may be managing certain aspects of their lives, for example working or looking after their family, going to college, but may be able to do little else.

For People Whose Activities Have Greatly Reduced

Initially, you may experience a slight increase in your symptoms when you start your activity program. However, this is usually only temporary, and occurs as a result of changing your 'usual' routine and increasing or introducing new activities. Once you become 'used' to your new routine your symptoms should gradually decrease.

For People Who Generally Do Too Much

Your symptoms should gradually decrease as you have more relaxation time. However, if you embark on new activities such as sport, or change your routine significantly, you may notice a temporary increase in your symptoms until you get more used to the activity/new routine.

For Everyone!

At times you may find the program difficult. This is understandable, because you may have been used to doing things when you felt like doing them, be it resting, sleeping, working, doing chores, and so on. As you will be aiming to do things at regular times, irrespective of how you are feeling, there may be times when you feel frustrated that you cannot do what you feel like doing. For example, sometimes you may feel like resting for longer than your program says, and at other times feel that you want to continue with a particular activity when the program you have written says that you are meant to be resting. These feelings are normal, but it is important that you do not succumb to them too often, as it may result in resuming old patterns of behavior that were unhelpful in the past. Persevere with your program, however difficult it may seem, and in time you will appreciate the benefits of gradually changing the way you do things.

Most people experience one or two minor setbacks (increased symptoms) when they are changing the way they do things. These may come about for a variety of reasons – you might have a viral infection, for example. Chapter 11 offers some guidelines on managing setbacks. Although these episodes can be irritating, they can also be a good opportunity to become an expert in managing difficult times.

Bear in mind that you can expect a temporary increase in your symptoms when you change your routine, increase your activities, and so on; so don't be disheartened if this happens. However, if you experience a sudden or severe increase in symptoms, or begin to experience distressing symptoms that you have not had before, you should consult your doctor.

An Outline of the Program Sequence

To give you an idea of the shape of the self-help program, we have suggested a sequence of steps to take you through the three core stages. This sequence is structured in a way that is often followed by people who attend sessions of cognitive behavior therapy with a therapist. It is not easy to give firm guidelines on how long each stage will take; you may, for example, feel that you need to spend longer on some parts and less time on others according to the severity and type of your own symptoms and how you progress.

The First Stage

As well as learning more about triggers and factors that may be maintaining your fatigue and how it affects you, we suggest that you do the following:

- *Complete activity diaries every day.* Keeping activity diaries will help you to monitor what you do in the daytime in terms of rest, work, chores, sleep, exercise, reading, etc.
- *Complete sleep diaries every day.* To find out more about your sleep pattern and how it could be improved, it can be useful

to keep a record of how long it takes you to get to sleep, whether you wake in the night, and whether your sleep pattern is very erratic.

- *Set targets.* This will give you clear goals to work towards and help you focus on what you would like to be doing in a few months from now. It is important that these targets are realistic and achievable.
- *Implement strategies to improve your sleep.* The strategies that you choose to implement will depend on what, if any, sleep-related problem you have identified.
- *Write an activity program to carry out every day.* After completing your activity and sleep diaries for a couple of weeks, you will have enough information to plan your first activity program. This program should include planned periods of both rest and various activities.

These initial parts of the self-help program are covered in Chapters 4–7.

The Middle Stage

Over a period of months, you will gradually work towards your long-term targets. This may involve increasing some existing activities, starting new ones, gathering more information about your condition and symptoms, reducing rests, and so on. In order for you to make as much progress as possible, we suggest that you do the following:

- *Review and change your activity program every couple of weeks.* Monitoring your progress at regular intervals will help you to focus on things that are going well and also on problem areas that may need more attention. What changes you make to your program will depend mainly on how successful you were in achieving your previous goals. In order to track your progress, it may help to keep up your activity and sleep diaries.
- *Work on unhelpful thoughts.* When you have established a good routine, with planned periods of activity and rest, you

37

will be in a position to look at any unhelpful thoughts that may hold back your progress. Chapter 8 aims to help you to identify and challenge unhelpful thoughts and beliefs that may be hampering your efforts to overcome your illness.

- *Address any other problems that are making it difficult for you to make progress.* As you start to feel better and become more active, you may come across other obstacles in the way of your progress. If this is the case, you may find it helpful to read and apply strategies from Chapter 9 ('Overcoming Blocks to Recovery') and Chapter 10 ('Overcoming Worry, Stress and Anxiety Related to Chronic Fatigue Syndrome').
- *Read about how to manage a setback and write a plan for this.* Chapter 11 identifies possible triggers for setbacks and discusses how to tackle them.

The Final Stage

We hope that by the time you have made some progress towards your targets and have established and maintained a good routine, containing a mixture of different activities and relaxation, you will be feeling a bit better, and will not need to monitor what you do quite so closely. However, before you reduce your diary-keeping, it is important that you give some thought to how to continue to make progress and how to manage a setback later, should one occur.

We recommend that you do the following:

- *Read Chapter 12, 'Case Studies'.* This review of a few other individuals' efforts and achievements will help you set your own work in context and give you some insight into the wider experience of CFS.
- *Read Chapter 13, 'Preparing for the Future'.* This chapter describes how you can sustain and build on your progress in order to reduce your fatigue and improve your well-being further.
- *Complete the 'Evaluation of progress' form in Chapter 13.* This will help you to check how much you have understood from

working through the book and will help you to identify any remaining areas of difficulty that you need to work on.

- *Write a plan for the next three months.* This will provide you with a focus and help you to work towards targets that you have not achieved yet, or to identify and work towards new ones.

Consolidation

We hope that, after working through the chapters of this book for a period of six to twelve months, your condition will have improved noticeably. Some readers may find that they are doing much of what they were doing before they developed fatigue. Others may feel that they still have some way to go. In order for you to make further progress, it will be important that you continue to evaluate your progress at regular intervals. We have included in Chapter 13 'Record of progress' forms for you to use to help you to keep on track in working towards your targets. You may also find it helpful from time to time to reread particular sections of the book.

4

Monitoring Activity, Rest and Sleep

This chapter describes how to monitor your waking and sleeping hours by keeping an activity diary in the daytime and a sleep diary for the night-time. Keeping these records is very important as they will highlight specific patterns that may be contributing to keeping your fatigue going.

Monitoring Your Activity Levels

In order for you to gain an accurate picture of how you spend each day, it is important that you record what you do in your activity diary every day.

For the first two weeks, you will use the diaries to form an accurate picture of exactly what you do each day. After a week or so, you may see a pattern emerging. For example, you may notice that you tend to be fairly active in the morning and rest all afternoon, or you may be busy during the week and do very little at the weekend. You may notice that you have short bursts of activity throughout the day, or you may not see any pattern at all.

After completing your activity diary for a couple of weeks, it is time to construct an activity program. The information from your activity diaries will help you to decide on how much rest and activity you should have each day. We show you how to build your activity program in Chapter 7.

What Do I Have to Do?

- Look at the three examples of completed activity diaries on pages 42–4.
- Using a photocopy of the blank activity diary on page 45, write down every day what you are doing at the times indicated in the left-most column.
- Include as much detail as possible about what you were doing and for how long.
- Complete your diaries for every hour of the day, however trivial the activity may seem.
- Record your activities at regular intervals throughout the day. If you leave it until the end of the day to fill in, the task may seem too overwhelming and you may forget some of the details.
- After completing your activity diaries for a couple of weeks or so, you will be ready to read Chapter 7 on 'Planning Activity and Rest'. This chapter will help you to create your first activity program.

Activity diary, example 1: A person who rests for most of the time

Week beginning.......................

Day	Monday	Tuesday	Wednesday	Thursday	Friday	Saturday	Sunday
Hours asleep last night	9 hours	10 hours	10½ hour	5 hours	9 hours	4¾ hours	7 hours
6–8 a.m.	Asleep	Asleep	Asleep	Asleep	Asleep	Woke at 6, dozed	Asleep
8–10 a.m.	Asleep	Woke at 9.30	Woke at 10	Woke at 8 in pain	Woke at 9.30	Breakfast in bed	Woke at 8.15 Bath
10–11 a.m.	Took a bath and had breakfast	Breakfast in bed	Bath and dressed	Stayed in bed	Bath and dressed	Stayed in bed until lunch	Dressed and had breakfast
11 a.m.–12 noon	Lay on the couch, resting	Washed face, brushed teeth	Doctor's appointment	Slept	Rested on couch	Dozing	Went to friend's house
12 noon–1 p.m.	Looked at paper	Lay on couch, read a letter	Home, exhausted	Mother brought up soup	Lunch	Dozing	Had lunch
1–2 p.m.	Lunch, made by Mum	Made toast and tea	To bed	Dozed	Shopping with mother by car	Dressed, had lunch	Watched a video
2–3 p.m.	Went to bed and slept	Went to bed	Slept	Went downstairs	Watched television	Relations round	Went home (by car)
3–4 p.m.	Slept	Dozed on and off	Tea and toast in bed	Watched television	Tidied up (10 mins)	→	Lay on couch
4–5 p.m.	Went downstairs and watched TV	Friend came round	Went downstairs	Phoned a friend	Went to bed, feeling poorly	→	Dozed
5–6 p.m.	→	→	Lay on couch	Went back to bed	Slept	Felt exhausted; dozed on couch	Dozed
6–7 p.m.	Ate evening meal	Friend left, exhausted	Had evening meal	Evening meal in bed	Slept	Slept	Had a bath
7–8 p.m.	Television	Had evening meal	Television	Listened to radio	Evening meal downstairs	Evening meal	Evening meal in bed
8 p.m.–12 midnight	Bed at 10.15	Bed at 8.30	Bed at 9.15	→	Watched television	Friend phoned; television	Dozed on and off
Time I went to sleep	1 a.m.	11 p.m.	2 a.m.	12 midnight	2 a.m.	1.30 a.m.	9 p.m.

42

Activity diary, example 2: A person who manages some activity, but quite erratically

Day	Monday	Tuesday	Wednesday	Thursday	Friday	Saturday	Sunday
Hours asleep last night	7 hours	8 hours	8½ hours	9 hours	6 hours	9½ hours	11 hours
6–8 a.m.	Woke at 8	Asleep	Asleep	Woke at 7, read in bed	Asleep	Asleep	Asleep
8–10 a.m.	Bath and dressed at 9	Up 8.45, bath and dressed	Dressed at 9.15, breakfast	Woke at 8, bath, dressed	Stayed in bed, felt rough	Got up at 10	Breakfast in bed
10–11 a.m.	Ate breakfast, washed up	Breakfast, tidied up	Walked to shops (15 mins)	Breakfast, cleared up	Slept	Bathed and dressed	Bath and dressed
11 a.m.–12 noon	Rested on couch	Bus to dentist	Unpacked shopping	Wrote a letter (½ hour)	Bath and dressed	Went to sister's house by train (1¼ hrs door to door)	Played with children
12 noon–1 p.m.	Lunch	Walked home (20 mins)	Lunch	Walked to post letter (10 mins)	Ate a sandwich	→	Went for a bar lunch
1–2 p.m.	Watched TV	Lunch	Rested on bed (dozing)	Lunch	Walked to shops (15 mins)	Played with sister's children	→
2–3 p.m.	Walked to shops (15 mins)	Slept on couch	→	Friend visited; chatted	Met friend, went to her house	Walk in the park (25 mins)	Walked in park (½ hr)
3–4 p.m.	Rested	→	Tidied my room	→	Listened to music	Fell asleep on couch	Train home
4–5 p.m.	Rested	Read for 15 mins	Read downstairs	Dozed on couch	Fell asleep	Helped to feed children	→
5–6 p.m.	Cooked and ate evening meal	Watched TV	Visited friends	Watched TV	Walked home (15 mins)	Read children a story	Fell asleep on couch
6–7 p.m.	Washed up, read (5 mins)	Prepared and ate evening meal	→	Cooked and ate evening meal	Heated a pre-packed meal	Had a take-out	Made a sandwich
7–8 p.m.	Listened to the radio	Washed up		Washed up	Ate evening meal and washed up	Chatted to sister	Went to bed and read
8 p.m.–12 midnight	Friend visited	Phoned friend. Bed at 9.15	Home, bed immediately	Bad headache, bed at 8.30	Watched TV	Went to bed at 11	
Time I went to sleep	12.30 a.m.	1.30 a.m.	10 p.m.	11 p.m.	11.30 p.m.	11.05 p.m.	9.30 p.m.

43

Activity diary, example 3: A person who is working, but is managing to do little at weekends or in the evenings

Week beginning...........................

Day	Monday	Tuesday	Wednesday	Thursday	Friday	Saturday	Sunday
Hours asleep last night	8 hours	7 hours	9 hours	6 hours	7 hours	11 hours	11 hours
6–8 a.m.	Woke at 8	Up 6.30. 2 hr drive to London	Asleep	Woke at 7, had shower	Up at 6.30	Asleep	Asleep
8–10 a.m.	Train to work	Breakfast, met clients	Woke at 8.30, had long bath	Train to work; paperwork	Train to work, then meetings	Asleep	Up at 9.45
10–11 a.m.	Meetings all morning	Met clients	Worked at home	Interviews all morning	Meetings	Asleep	Played with children
11 a.m.–12 noon	→	Meetings for most of the day	→	→	→	Got up at 11.30	Did some gardening
12 noon–1 p.m.	→	→	→	→	→	Lunch	Went to lunch with friends
1–2 p.m.	Lunch at desk (10 mins)	Lunch at restaurant	→	Lunch at desk	Lunch out with colleagues	Watched sport on TV	→
2–3 p.m.	Paperwork and phone calls	→	Train to work	Paperwork and phone calls	→	→	→
3–4 p.m.	→	→	Paperwork	→	Paperwork	→	Home, fell asleep
4–5 p.m.	→	→	Phone calls	→	Phone calls	Helped feed children	→
5–6 p.m.	→	Drove home, took 3 hours	Meeting	Home, read to children	Train home	Read children a story	Prepared for meeting Monday
6–7 p.m.	Train home; phone calls	→	→	Long relaxing bath	Friends round for evening meal	Fell asleep	Long relaxing bath
7–8 p.m.	Evening meal	Evening meal	Took clients out for a meal	Evening meal	→	Evening meal	Evening meal
8 p.m.–12 midnight	Watched TV. Bed at 10	Fell asleep at about 8.30	Home at 11.30	Work for tomorrow	Bed at midnight	Watched a video	More work. Bed at 11
Time I went to sleep	10.30 p.m.	8.30 p.m.	1 a.m.	1 a.m.	12.30 p.m.	11 p.m.	12 midnight

44

Activity diary

Day	Monday	Tuesday	Wednesday	Thursday	Friday	Saturday	Sunday
Hours asleep last night							
6–8 a.m.							
8–10 a.m.							
10–11 a.m.							
11 a.m.–12 noon							
12 noon–1 p.m.							
1–2 p.m.							
2–3 p.m.							
3–4 p.m.							
4–5 p.m.							
5–6 p.m.							
6–7 p.m.							
7–8 p.m.							
8 p.m.–12 midnight							
Time I went to sleep							

Monitoring Your Sleep Pattern

To help you to build up an accurate picture of how you sleep, complete a sleep diary for two weeks, in addition to recording your activities and rest periods during the daytime in your activity diary. This will help you to see at a glance what your sleep pattern is like and whether there is anything that you would like to change. For example, you may notice that on a number of nights it takes you a while to get to sleep, that you get up at very different times each day, or that you wake frequently in the night.

What Do I Have To Do?

- Look at the example of a completed sleep diary on page 47.
- Using a photocopy of the blank sleep diary on page 48, complete your sleep diary when you wake up in the morning for at least two weeks.
- After completing your sleep diary for two weeks, you will be ready to turn to page 59 and read Chapter 6, which outlines and explains techniques to help you to improve your sleep.
- Decide what you would like to change about your sleep pattern and, when you come to construct your first activity program (Chapter 7), write down the strategies that would help you to achieve your aims.
- You may find it helpful to continue to monitor your sleep for a few more weeks to see if your sleep improves as a result of implementing some of the strategies.

Example of a completed sleep diary

	Monday	Tuesday	Wednesday	Thursday	Friday	Saturday	Sunday
Last night I went to bed at . . . and turned the lights out at . . .	9.15 p.m. 10 p.m.	9.30 p.m. 9.45 p.m.	10 p.m. 10.30 p.m.	9.45 p.m. 10.15 p.m.	11 p.m. 11 p.m.	12.30 a.m. 12.30 a.m.	9.30 p.m. 9.45 p.m.
After turning out the lights, I fell asleep in . . . (estimate)	30 mins	Straight away	Straight away	1 hour	5–10 mins	Straight away	About 2 hours
I woke up . . . times in the night	1	0	0	2	0	1	2
On each waking during the night, I was awake for . . . (estimate)	2 mins	–	–	5 mins 30 mins	–	5 mins	15 mins 30 mins
I woke up at . . . (time of last waking)	With alarm at 8 a.m.	7.30 a.m.	8 a.m. with alarm	9.30 a.m.	8 a.m. with alarm	10 a.m.	8.30 a.m.
I got out of bed for the day at . . .	8.30 a.m.	8 a.m.	8.15 a.m.	10 a.m.	8.15 a.m.	10.30 a.m.	9 a.m.
Overall, my sleep last night was . . . (0 = very sound, 8 = very restless)	2	0	0	5	0	2	2
When I got up this morning I felt . . . (0 = refreshed, 8 = exhausted)	5	4	4	6	3	5	6
Comments/reasons for a good or a particularly bad night				Felt hot and achy	Better night: bath before bed relaxed me		Worrying about new job tomorrow

47

Sleep diary

	Monday	Tuesday	Wednesday	Thursday	Friday	Saturday	Sunday
Last night I went to bed at . . . and turned the lights out at . . .							
After turning out the lights, I fell asleep in . . . mins/hrs (estimate)							
I woke up . . . times in the night							
On each waking during the night, I was awake for . . . mins (estimate)							
I woke up at . . . (time of last waking)							
I got out of bed for the day at . . .							
Overall, my sleep last night was . . . . (0=very sound, 8=very restless)							
When I got up this morning I felt . . . (0=refreshed, 8=exhausted)							
Comments/reasons for a good or a particularly bad night							

5

Setting Targets

Setting targets is an important step in helping you to overcome your chronic fatigue problems. In the past you may have prioritized just a few activities such as professional or income-earning work, housework, and/or looking after the family, and may have neglected time for yourself – your hobbies, time to see your friends, and so on. Setting targets will therefore give you the opportunity to develop a more balanced lifestyle, and this in turn can contribute to reducing your fatigue.

When Would Be a Good Time to Plan My Targets?

We suggest that you plan your targets after a couple of weeks of completing your activity and sleep diaries. You will then have had the opportunity to identify areas of your life that you would like to change.

Important Facts about Targets

- Targets are things that you would like to be doing in the longer term, rather than something you want to achieve immediately.
- Set yourself a range of *different* types of target to work towards to make your life as balanced as possible. So, rather than addressing one particular area of your life, e.g. work, try to ensure that your targets contain a *mixture* of activities.

- Remember that pleasurable activities are as important as income-earning work, household chores, etc.
- Set yourself *realistic* and *achievable* targets. So be wary of being too 'driven' or 'ambition-orientated' when setting your targets. For example, if you have not worked for several years, it would be better to set yourself a target of taking up voluntary or part-time work, rather than a full-time job. Or, if you have not walked for a long time, it would be better to set a target of walking for 15 minutes a day rather than walking for an hour at a time. Remember that you will be able to change your targets once your initial ones have been achieved; so you don't have to bite off more than you can chew at the first attempt.
- Make your targets *specific*, in terms of:
  - *what it is* you want to do (activity);
  - *how often* you would like to carry out the activity (frequency);
  - the *length of time* to be spent on the activity (duration).
- Although you may feel that your choice of targets is very restricted because of your symptoms, setting targets, however modest, will provide you with a clear direction and focus.

How to Set Targets

- Look at the examples of target areas on the next page to get some ideas for your targets.
- Write a list of things that you would like to work towards over the coming months.
- Divide your list into target areas (e.g. work, social, exercise, leisure).
- Look at the examples of targets on page 52, to ensure that your targets are clearly defined and specific.
- Choose at least four targets and complete a target breakdown sheet for each of them, as described on page 53 in the section on 'How To Break Down Your Targets into Manageable Steps'. Blank sheets are provided on pages 56–8.

Examples of Target Areas

Leisure Time

You may find that your time at home is taken up with chores. Think about planning regular time for pleasurable activities; for example, reading, playing a musical instrument, painting, writing letters, 'quality time' with children or partner. There may be hobbies you have neglected – or you may have always had a burning desire to try something new!

Work/Education

If you are *not* working, you may consider going back to your old job (if applicable), doing part-time work, or doing some voluntary work.

If you *are* working, you may feel that you are working excessively, and would benefit from reducing your hours.

You may consider some type of educational course to enable you to find work or change direction in your career, or simply because you have an interest in a particular subject. The material in Chapter 14 on work, courses, and resources (see pages 184–92) may provide you with some useful leads.

Social Activities

There may be friends and family with whom you have lost touch, or whom you see only rarely. You may like to consider making a regular time for talking to/meeting up with those people. Alternatively, you may like to explore options for meeting new people.

Exercise

In the past you may have exercised regularly. On the other hand, you may never have been particularly fit and have had exercise on a 'to do' list for many years. You may like to consider setting aside time for a particular type of exercise.

Chores/DIY/Gardening

You may have been unable to do much in your home or garden for some time because of your fatigue; if this is the case, you may feel that you would like to aim at doing some home improvements or a gardening project. Or you may feel that you are endlessly doing chores and could benefit from allocating a specific time to spend on them rather than having them always hanging over you.

Sleep

If sleep is a big problem, you may choose to focus on a specific target in relation to this; for example, a regular getting up time, or not sleeping in the day.

Examples of Targets

Be sure to make your targets specific and clearly defined.

Examples of Clearly Defined Targets

- To go shopping twice a week for half an hour.
- To have a friend for coffee once a week for half an hour.
- To walk for 15 minutes daily.
- To do voluntary work three times a week for at least two hours on each occasion.
- To go out with friends once a week for up to three hours.
- To swim twice weekly for half an hour on each occasion.
- To do a course at college for three hours weekly.
- To do gardening three times a week for half an hour.
- To spend one hour daily on my hobby (specify the hobby).
- To do one hour of chores daily; e.g. ironing, washing, cleaning.
- To work part-time in the profession for which I am trained.
- To have two breaks at work of at least 15 minutes each, daily.
- To sit and read the paper/a magazine for half an hour daily.

- To get up by 9 a.m. each day.
- To stay out of bed until 10 p.m. each night.

These are all measurable targets, so you will know when you have achieved them.

Examples of Not Clearly Defined Targets

- To go to work. (No frequency or duration specified.)
- To go out socially more often. (No frequency or duration specified.)
- To be more active. (No activity, frequency or duration specified.)
- To feel better. (No activity, frequency or duration specified.)

These are just vague ideas and not measurable; you would therefore *not* know when you had met them, and would risk feeling uncertain, frustrated and discouraged.

How to Break Down Your Targets into Manageable Steps

As we have already mentioned, targets are things that you want to achieve in the longer term. Therefore, in order to work towards them in a way that you will be able to monitor and assess, you will need to break down each one into manageable steps. You can then gradually introduce the consecutive steps into your activity program.

- Look at the examples overleaf that have been broken down into manageable steps.
- Think of ways to break down each of your own targets into manageable steps.
- Make each step small, and grade it from easy to difficult.
- Write down your steps to achieving your targets on your target breakdown sheets (see pages 56–8 for some blank sheets).

Examples of Breaking Down Targets into Manageable Steps

Target: To go for two ten-minute walks every day.

Steps to achieving target:
- To get out of bed/up from my chair each hour and walk round the room.
- To walk round my house for one minute every hour.
- To walk round the garden/house for two minutes each hour.
- To go for three three-minute walks every day.
- To go for three five-minute walks every day.
- To go for two seven-minute walks every day.
- To go for two ten-minute walks every day.

Target: To go out with friends once a week for up to three hours.

Steps to achieving target:
- To talk to a friend on the phone for 15 minutes three times a week.
- To go to a friend who lives close by for half an hour once a week.
- To go to a friend who lives close by for an hour once a week.
- To go out with a friend to a local venue for an hour once a week.
- To go out with friend(s) for one and a half hours a week.
- To go out with friend(s) for two hours a week.
- To go out with friend(s) for two and a half hours a week.
- To go out with friend(s) for three hours a week.

Target: To read for half an hour, twice a day.

Steps to achieving target:
- To read for 15 minutes, twice a day.
- To read for 20 minutes, twice a day.
- To read for 30 minutes, twice a day.

Target: To do voluntary work three times a week for at least two hours on each occasion.

Steps to achieving target:
- To write a list of kinds of voluntary work in which I am interested.
- To contact the appropriate association(s) for information.
- To plan steps which will help me *sustain* the activity in which I want to be involved; e.g. standing for longer periods (if working in a charity shop), reading/computer work (if doing administrative work), etc.
- Arrange informal visit(s) to the workplace.
- Arrange a graded work schedule if possible; e.g.
    one hour twice weekly for a couple of weeks; then
    one hour three times a week; then
    two hours three times a week.

Target: To do something relaxing for myself for one hour every day.

Steps to achieving target:
- To leave work on time each day.
- To ask other family members to help with the chores.
- To make a list of non-urgent tasks that can be put off to another day.
- To plan a list of pleasurable things that I would like to do each day.
- To choose one of these each day and spend an hour on it.

You may only need two or three steps to achieve a target, or you may need a lot more. We have included space on each target breakdown sheet for two targets, with eight steps to each. Use extra paper if there is not enough space on the sheets for all the steps you want to include.

Target breakdown sheet

TARGET   STEPS TO ACHIEVING TARGET

1

2

3

4

5

6

7

8

TARGET   STEPS TO ACHIEVING TARGET

1

2

3

4

5

6

7

8

Target breakdown sheet

TARGET   STEPS TO ACHIEVING TARGET

1

2

3

4

5

6

7

8

TARGET   STEPS TO ACHIEVING TARGET

1

2

3

4

5

6

7

8

Target breakdown sheet

TARGET   STEPS TO ACHIEVING TARGET

1

2

3

4

5

6

7

8

TARGET   STEPS TO ACHIEVING TARGET

1

2

3

4

5

6

7

8

Improving Your Sleep

Sleep problems in people with chronic fatigue syndrome are very common. Difficulties include:

- taking a long time to go to sleep at night;
- waking frequently and/or staying awake during the night;
- waking early;
- sleeping too much.

The quality of sleep is often poor and sufferers will often report waking up feeling exhausted.

This chapter aims to help you to identify some of the things that may be contributing to your sleep problems, and offers strategies to overcome each problem.

When Would Be a Good Time to Implement the Suggested Strategies?

After you have been keeping your sleep diary for a couple of weeks you will have identified your own sleep problems. You can then start to implement the relevant strategies. Most people find it easier to do this gradually; however, a few individuals have reported that 'short, sharp shock' treatment works best for them. We suggest that you limit the number of changes you make to those that you can carry out regularly. So, for example, if you stay in bed until lunchtime every day, and have a nap in the afternoon, and go to bed in the early evening, you may find it easier to start by gradually getting up earlier and cutting out the nap, while leaving your bedtime the same. Write down the strategies that you intend to use on your activity program.

Lifestyle and Environmental Factors That Contribute to Poor Sleep

- An *irregular sleep pattern* can disrupt the body clock and lead to the loss of certain cues, such as feeling tired in the evening and alert in the morning.
- *Daytime inactivity* can increase your feeling of fatigue and desire for catnaps.
- *Sleeping in the day* will lead you to need less sleep at night.
- *Alcohol and other substances,* such as caffeine-containing drinks (coffee, tea, cola), cigarettes, and certain medications can make it difficult to go to sleep and/or wake you up in the night.
- An *uncomfortable sleeping environment,* such as an uncomfortable mattress, being too hot or cold, a restless partner, or excessive noise may keep you awake at night. Studying or doing other paperwork in your bedroom may make it more difficult for you to 'switch off' at night. Long periods of wakefulness in your bed may lead you to associate your room or bed with being awake, therefore making it more difficult for you to go to sleep.
- An *overly active mind or worries at bedtime* can lead to tension, restlessness, and an inability to relax, again making it more difficult to fall asleep.
- *Sleeping too much* can make you feel constantly tired, as the sleep is often 'light' and non-refreshing.

Strategies to Improve Your Sleep

You may find that your sleep will improve once you increase your level of activity slightly, as described in Chapter 7. On the other hand, you may need to follow some of the methods described below for a few weeks or even months before you notice any significant changes.

Establish a Routine

The aim of establishing a routine is to help your body clock to get used to certain things happening at set times. This will help to regulate your body (circadian) rhythms, so that you begin to 'feel' things at certain times each day and establish a regular sleep–wake cycle. We do not recommend that you should start out by going to bed at the same time every evening, as you may not feel sleepy at that time. However, you may find that when you start getting up at the same time each day you get more tired at a particular time of the evening, and therefore naturally start going to bed at a similar time each day.

The guidelines below will help you to establish a routine. If your sleep pattern is very erratic, you may find it difficult to put them into practice all at once.

In order to establish a routine:

- *Get up at the same time each day*, even if you have not had much sleep the previous night. It may be helpful to set your alarm clock.
- *Do not nap during the day*, even if you feel very tired; or, if this is too difficult, gradually reduce the length of the nap.
- *Try not to go to bed early*, even if you feel very tired, or to make up for lost sleep. You may find it helpful to set a time before which you will *not* go to bed.

Associate Your Bed and Bedroom with Sleep Rather than Being Awake

If you have slept badly for a long time, you may find that when you get into bed, instead of feeling sleepy, you feel wide awake or restless, and cannot easily fall asleep. Subconsciously, you may therefore associate your bed/bedroom with being awake rather than being asleep, and this itself may make it harder to fall asleep.

The following guidelines aim to help you to associate your bed and bedroom with sleep rather than wakefulness.

- Avoid using your bedroom during the day if at all possible. If you live in a one-room apartment, or one room in a house or student accommodation, try to have a separate work area in your room, so that you just use your bed for sleep.
- Your bed should be for sleep and (if applicable) sex only. So don't read, study, watch television, or sort out the day's problems in bed, as these are waking activities. (If this is difficult for you, see 'Problem-Solving Strategy for Reducing Worries at Night' on pages 65–6.)
- Go to bed when you are sleepy, rather than at a time you think you should go. For example, if you think that you should go to bed at about 11.00 p.m., but do not feel sleepy, wait until you feel sleepy.
- Do not be tempted to go to bed very early (e.g. before 9.30 p.m.), even if you feel very sleepy, as you may wake in the middle of the night or early in the morning.
- Turn the light off straight away when you get into bed.
- If you are not asleep within 20 minutes, go to another room and sit and relax or read until you feel sleepy again.
- Repeat the previous step as often as is required, and also if you wake up for periods of more than about 20 minutes in the night.

Try to follow this program rigidly. It can take several weeks, or even months, to establish an efficient and regular pattern. If you have a partner, you may like to discuss with them ways to help you to keep to these guidelines as best you can. This may involve some compromises for both of you.

Establish an Optimal Sleep Pattern

An optimal sleep pattern is one in which you fall asleep within a short time of going to bed, have good-quality sleep, and wake seldom and briefly during the night.

Your sleep pattern is *optimal* when it is both *efficient* and *regular*. When you are asleep for the greater proportion of the time you spend in bed, the more *efficient* your sleep is. The more closely one night's time in bed and time asleep resemble other nights', the more *regular* your sleep is. To establish your optimal sleep pattern, you will reduce the amount of time you are in bed in order to increase the amount of time you are asleep. This can be done in conjunction with the guidelines in the above two sections, or separately.

- Calculate your *total* time asleep on an 'average' night.
- Stay in bed only for the time that you are usually asleep. For example, if you are usually in bed for ten hours a night, but asleep for only seven and a half hours in total, you should stay in bed for only seven and a half hours.
- You may feel more tired for a while, but the slight sleep deprivation you may experience will in turn lead to your going to sleep more quickly, waking up less often, sleeping more deeply.
- The time in bed can be gradually increased as your sleep efficiency improves (if applicable).

If You Sleep Too Much, Reduce Your Sleep at Night

Sleeping for longer than you used to before having CFS may contribute to feelings of exhaustion in the morning. If you sleep for more than about an hour longer than you did prior to having CFS, you may feel better if you reduce the amount of time you sleep at night.

- Cut down your sleep time gradually, either by going to bed half an hour later or by getting up half an hour earlier.
- Establish set times for getting up and going to bed.
- Be consistent in either getting up earlier or going to bed later.
- Do not compensate by getting up later or going to bed earlier, even if you feel more tired.

- Review your sleep pattern weekly, and continue to reduce your sleep time gradually until you are more 'refreshed' on waking.

You may feel more tired for the first few weeks after changing your sleep routine, but in the long run you can expect the quality of your sleep to increase as the quantity of your sleep decreases.

Improve Your Sleep Hygiene

'Sleep hygiene' refers to lifestyle and environmental factors that may be beneficial or detrimental to sleep.
The following guidelines may help to promote an improved sleep pattern.

- *Exercise:* Avoid exercise within three hours of bedtime, as this may wake you up. Exercise in the late afternoon may deepen sleep at night.
- *Diet:* A light snack before bedtime may be sleep inducing, but a heavy meal too close to bedtime will interfere with sleep. Fluid intake should be limited.
- *Caffeine* stimulates the central nervous system; it is associated with delaying sleep onset and can cause wakefulness. Substances containing caffeine, e.g. coffee, tea, chocolate, and cola, should be avoided for four to six hours before bedtime and during the night if you wake up. Coffee generally contains about twice as much caffeine as other caffeinated drinks.
- *Nicotine* also stimulates the central nervous system, and although many people say that cigarettes help them to relax, the overall effect is one of stimulation rather than relaxation. Smoking cigarettes should therefore be avoided near bedtime and if you waken in the night.
- *Alcohol* depresses the central nervous system. Although it may help you drop off to sleep, it often causes disrupted sleep later in the night as it is metabolized. It is unusual for people

with CFS to drink much alcohol but, if you do, it is best avoided in the hours before bedtime. A milky drink before bed can help you to feel sleepy and will not cause you to waken in the night.

- *Environment:* Your bed and mattress should be comfortable. Keep light and noise to a minimum during your sleep period. Don't keep your bedroom too hot – it should be around 18 °C. Use window blinds if necessary, earplugs if you live in a particularly noisy place and are unable to get used to it, and a fan or heater to control temperature.

Preparing for Sleep

Establishing a set routine will help you to prepare both mentally and physically for going to sleep.

- Try to wind down in the hour or so before you go to bed.
- Include relaxing activities such as watching television, having a warm bath, listening to music in your 'winding-down' schedule.
- Avoid stimulating activities which will keep you alert; e.g. work, studying, decision making.
- Develop a regular order of doing things; e.g. locking up the house, turning out the lights, brushing your teeth. This will act as a signal to your body that it is preparing for sleep.

Problem-Solving Strategy for Reducing Worries at Night

Lying in bed at night worrying about problems can make you feel tense and prevent you from going to sleep. The strategy described below may help you to avoid worrying at night, enabling you to feel more relaxed and get to sleep more quickly:

- Set aside 20 minutes in the early evening.
- Use this time to write down problems or loose ends that you have not dealt with during the day.

- Write down possible steps to resolve the problems or to tie up the loose ends.
- Allocate time to do the actual work.
- Also consider other, longer-term problems which may intrude on your sleep; e.g. emotional, financial, or other worries.
- For each of these, write down the first or next positive step of action to take, and when you will take it.
- If you cannot go to sleep or wake up worrying about a problem, remind yourself that you have the matter in hand and that worrying about it now will not help.
- If new worries occur to you at night, write them down on a notepad or a piece of paper, and 'deal' with them the next day, in the same way.
- You may also find it helpful to refer to Chapter 10 on 'Overcoming Worry, Stress and Anxiety', and Chapter 8 on 'Overcoming Unhelpful Thinking Patterns'.

How to Deal with Frustration about Not Being Able to Sleep

If you become frustrated about not being able to fall asleep, and worry about the possible 'negative' consequences the next day, it is likely that you will inhibit sleep further by trying harder to fall asleep. So:

- Do not try too hard to fall asleep.
- Tell yourself that 'sleep will come when it is ready', and that 'relaxing in bed is almost as good as being asleep'.
- Try to keep your eyes open in the darkened room, and as they (naturally) try to close, tell yourself to resist closing them for another few seconds. This procedure 'tempts' sleep to take over.
- Visualize a pleasing scene, or try repeating a neutral word (such as 'the') every few seconds.

Planning Activity and Rest

One of the most important strategies in overcoming your fatigue problems will be to learn how to construct your own program of planned activity and rest. This chapter will help you first to develop a better routine, and then to work towards the targets you set yourself in working through Chapter 5. At the end of the chapter we discuss the possibility of your using a different kind of record, called a Target Achievement Record, to monitor your activities when you feel that you have developed a good routine. The target achievement record takes less time to complete than the activity diary, and some people who have used it prefer it.

When Can I Plan My First Activity Program?

You can plan your first activity program as soon as you feel that you have a clear idea of your overall pattern of activity and rest in the day, and your pattern of sleep at night. This will probably be at least two weeks after starting to complete your diaries. The aim of your first activity program will be to stabilize what you are already doing rather than to make any big changes.

Different Programs for Different Circumstances

Because chronic fatigue syndrome affects people in such diverse ways, we have separated this chapter into two sections. Although you are likely to find one section more applicable to your own circumstances than the other, you may want to read them both.

- *Section 1 is for people whose activities have greatly reduced.* This section aims to help people who have significantly cut down all or most of the things they used to do before they had CFS. (See below.)
- *Section 2 is for people who generally do too much.* This section aims to help people who are able to manage certain aspects of their lives, such as work, but feel so exhausted that they are unable to do much else. (Please turn to page 76.)

SECTION 1: PLANNING ACTIVITY AND REST FOR PEOPLE WHOSE ACTIVITIES HAVE GREATLY REDUCED

We have already discussed the factors that frequently contribute to the maintenance of chronic fatigue syndrome. We hope that by now you will have a better understanding of some of the things that are responsible for keeping your own CFS going, like a poor sleep pattern, doing things in bursts, or resting for long periods.

Although you will probably have tried a variety of things to help you feel better, you may feel that you are taking two steps forward and one step back.

A very common factor that contributes to the maintenance of CFS is reduced activity and increased rest. As we explained in Chapter 1, reduced or irregular activity and prolonged periods of rest cause physical changes in the body. These changes cause unpleasant sensations and symptoms that can be very distressing and often lead people to have an erratic pattern of rest and activity dependent on how they feel.

Your symptoms may be so severe that you spend much of your time confined to bed or a chair, and your days and nights run into each other. You may find that *any* activity is exhausting: brushing your hair, talking, walking around a room, getting dressed or washed. On the other hand, you may find that you can be reasonably active on some days, but as a result of 'doing too much' you then become more fatigued and find that other symptoms increase, so that you cannot do very much on other days.

We all need adequate rest to be healthy. People with CFS often find that they rest more than they used to, but rarely find themselves more refreshed as a result. This may be for the following reasons:

- Your body does not get a chance to get used to a regular routine, as you may be resting in response to your symptoms of fatigue and pain, rather than in a planned way.
- Although you probably *feel* that you need more rest, too much rest can be counterproductive as it may lead to disturbed sleep and reduced physical fitness; in fact, it can make you feel *more* tired and lethargic.
- It may be difficult for you to relax properly, as you may find it hard to 'switch off' when you try to rest; e.g. you may be thinking about all the jobs that you need to do.

In order to establish a better balance of activity and rest, it is important to plan in advance what you are going to do each day: this is what you will be doing in creating an 'activity program'.

Important Facts to Consider When Planning an Activity Program

- The key to becoming more active is to aim for *consistency* and *regularity* in both activity and rest, regardless of how you feel. It is important that you plan small chunks of activity at regular intervals, rather than long periods of occasional activity. As you increase your level of everyday activities you will gradually become stronger and be able to cut down on rest.
- Try to plan to do about the same amount of activity, and have the same number of rests, each day. This may be difficult due to practical restraints such as work or childcare commitments, but aim for as much consistency as possible.

- When writing your first activity program, aim for about as much 'overall' activity as you are having at present. So, for example, if you do all your cleaning on one day and it takes you two hours, break it down into four half-hourly chunks spread throughout the week.
- It is important to think about what you will do during your rest time. Rests are a time for you to try to relax. What you do in your rest time will depend on your level of fatigue and the things that you find relaxing. Some people may find that reading is relaxing; for others, reading may be a major activity. Listening to the radio or music, or watching television, are other relaxing things you may consider. The important thing is that the rest time is used as a break from activity.
- Try to avoid using your bed for resting or sleeping during the day, however tired you feel. Sleeping in the day or resting in your bedroom is likely to affect your sleep at night.

Refer to your target breakdown sheet on pages 56–8 for guidance on some of the activities that you may like to include in your activity program.

Steps to Creating an Activity Program

Planning Activities

- Write a list of activities that you would like to do during the next week on your activity program. (Examples can be found on pages 79–80 and a blank activity program is provided on page 82.) For each activity, specify how often you want to do it and how long you want to spend on it on each occasion: e.g. 'talk to a friend for 15 minutes every other day', 'read for half an hour every day'.
- Use your activity diaries for guidance on the time to be spent on each activity during the week to make sure you don't overdo it.
- Remember to make your activity times manageable chunks, rather than one long session; e.g. if you have been doing one

solid hour of housework each day, divide it into three chunks of 20 minutes each.
- Remember to include strategies to improve your sleep.

Planning Rests

- Look at the activity diaries that you have completed and estimate the average amount of rest taken each day.
- Write down on your activity program the number of rests to be taken each day, and the length of each rest.

For example, you might specify three one-hour rests every day, or two half-hour rests, or eight rests of 45 minutes.

You can use the formula below to calculate your initial amount of resting time.

- Look at your activity diaries and add up the total number of hours of rest that you have had during the period in which you completed them; e.g. if you have completed your diaries for 14 days, add up the times you have spent resting during those days.
- Divide the number of hours of rest by the number of days you have completed your diaries: this will give you an estimate of the amount of rest that you should have each day.

Example:

Total rest over 14 days = 42 hours

$42 \div 14 = 3$

Amount of rest to be taken each day: 3 hours.

Example of an Initial Activity Program

For someone who is resting for about three hours a day:
- To get up and get dressed by 8 a.m.
- To have three one-hour rests in a chair (e.g. at 10 a.m., 2 p.m., and 6 p.m.) every day.

- To go for three ten-minute walks every day.
- To read for 20 minutes every day.
- To do chores for half an hour twice a day.
- To talk to friends on the phone for 15 minutes a day.
- To go to bed by 11.00 p.m.

For someone who is resting for about six hours a day:
- To get up and get dressed by 9.00 a.m.
- To go for two ten-minute walks every day.
- To do chores for 15 minutes four times a day.
- To talk to friends on the phone for ten minutes, three times a week.
- To read for ten minutes twice a day.
- To rest in a chair for six one-hour periods, evenly spaced throughout the day.
- To go to bed after 10.30 p.m.

For someone who is resting for most of the day:
- To get out of bed by 9.00 a.m.
- To walk around the house for one minute each hour.
- To rest for 50 minutes each hour.
- To do some activity (specify what) for ten minutes each hour,
    - e.g.   get washed and brush teeth by 9.30 a.m. every day;
      get dressed by 10.30 a.m. every day;
      read for 10 minutes twice every day;
      wash and dry dishes twice a day.

Recording Your Activities

You will already be used to recording your activities in your activity diary. It is important that you continue to write down what you are doing for each hour of the day in your activity diary as you begin your activity program, so that you can monitor your progress.

What to Expect When You Start Your Activity Program

As we mentioned earlier, your symptoms may increase slightly when you start your activity program. However, this is generally temporary and occurs as a result of changing your usual routine. Even though you may feel like resting more, it is important that you keep going with your activity program. It is usually the case that your symptoms will gradually decrease, although this may take a few weeks, sometimes longer.

Increasing Your Activity Levels

Once you have established a more consistent pattern of activity and rest, you will be in a position to start to increase – *gradually* – the amount of activity you do each day. This will probably be about two weeks after you start your activity program. By this time, we would hope that you will feel that you are managing your planned activities and planned rests fairly consistently.

- Look at your activity program and ask yourself, for each different activity: 'How successful was I at completing it?'
- Using Table 7.1 overleaf to guide you, set new levels for each of your activities.

How Often Should I Make Changes to My Activity Program?

How often you change your activity program will depend on how successful you are in achieving your plans. However, we would recommend that you set aside 15–30 minutes each week to review your activity program. This will give you the opportunity to assess your progress and help you to decide whether you can make any changes to your activity program for the next week. We recommend that you make at least one revision a month.

Table 7.1 **Increasing activity levels**

Success in achieving activity 0% = no success 100% = complete success	Possible reasons for achievement/ non-achievement	How to change your activity level/program
0–25%	Activity level set much too high; an acute illness	Reduce the level of those activities that you did not achieve on a regular basis*
	Other factors; e.g. moving house, holidays, other commitments getting in the way	Keep activity levels the same, or reduce only slightly
25–50%	Activity level may have been set slightly too high	Reduce your activity level slightly if nearer 25% achievement level; otherwise keep activity level the same
50–75%	Activity level set about right	Keep your activity level the same if nearer the 50% achievement level; otherwise slightly increase the activity level**
75–100%	Activity level set about right	Increase** your activity level, unless you have reached your target, in which case keep the activity level the same

*For example, if you planned to cook a meal once a day and did not manage to do so at all, maybe plan to cook a meal just twice a week. Or if you planned to get up at 9 a.m. every day and managed to do so only once, maybe reset getting-up time at 9.15 a.m.

**The amount of time by which you increase your activity will depend on what the activity is and the time that you are already spending on it. For guidance, please refer to Chapter 5 on setting targets.

When Should I Introduce New Activities?

You may consider introducing new activities:

- *When the overall success of the previous week's/fortnight's activity program reaches about 75 per cent.* It is important that you feel that you are managing your program reasonably well before adding in new activities. Otherwise you may end up feeling a little out of control.
- *When you have achieved a target.* When you have achieved one of your targets, you may find that you have the time to introduce another activity. So, for example, if you have achieved a target of going out socially once a week, you may feel like adding a new social activity each week or perhaps doing something different, such as a regular exercise class or evening class.
- *If, for reasons beyond your control, you are unable to continue to work towards a particular target.* Sometimes you will find that you plan targets that are not manageable for a variety of reasons. So, for example, if one of your targets was to go swimming each week and the pool was closed for cleaning, you might substitute another exercise for swimming. If you have planned a target to send emails for 15 minutes three times a week and your computer breaks down, plan to write to friends instead.
- *When your rests have decreased and you have the time for more activities.* Once you reduce your resting time you will be able to include another activity or to increase one that you are already doing. So, for example, if one of your rests used to last for one hour and is now half an hour, you can use that time to include another activity.
- It is *not* necessary for your fatigue to have decreased for you to increase or start a new activity.

How Do I Decrease My Rests?

Once your program has been established for a few weeks you are likely to have recovered from any temporary increase in fatigue and feel that you are able to reduce your rests. Gradually cut down the *amount* of time you spend resting at first. So, for example, if you rest for an hour three times a day, you may start by reducing each rest by ten minutes. Or, if you rest for half an hour six times a day, you may want to reduce three of the rests by five minutes and leave the others at half an hour.

If you have a lot of rest periods in the day, say, more than five, you may want to reduce the *number* of rests once you have reduced the amount of time resting.

If you find yourself feeling much better you should continue to include some short rests in the day; otherwise you may get into the cycle of pushing yourself too hard for too long and having to take long 'recovery' rests. We would recommend that you have at least a mid-morning and a mid-afternoon break, as well as one at lunchtime.

SECTION 2: PLANNING ACTIVITY AND REST FOR PEOPLE WHO GENERALLY DO TOO MUCH

We have already discussed the factors that frequently contribute to the maintenance of chronic fatigue syndrome. We hope that by now you will have a better understanding of some of the things that are responsible for keeping your own CFS going, such as keeping on the go all day without a break and/or sleeping erratically.

People who generally do too much are often able to 'keep going' at work, maintain their home, or study for long periods, but in the evenings and at weekends spend most of their time resting or sleeping in an attempt to feel better. This pattern can be very frustrating, causing you to miss out on pleasurable activities such as seeing friends or family, taking days out, doing some exercise, or pursuing your hobbies.

The key to improving your health is to make your life as balanced as possible. It is therefore important that you identify areas that you could change. For example, do you find that you tend to keep going at work without taking breaks? Do you find that you do not sit down at home until you have taken your children to school, tidied the house, and done the shopping? Do you find that you do not leave work until you have completed everything there is to do, even if it is late? Do you study for hours without taking a break and then have to sleep for a couple of days because you feel so fatigued? If the answer to some of the above questions is yes, then maybe you could consider some of the following ideas.

- Could you leave work a little earlier?
- Could you have a proper lunch break, instead of eating a sandwich at your desk?
- Could you postpone the cleaning, washing, preparing meals, and so on, and sit down for half an hour?
- Could you plan one or two pleasurable activities each week?
- Could you put aside one hour for yourself each day?
- Could you break up your studies with a brisk walk?

It is important to plan in advance what you are going to do each day by creating an activity program once a week. This will help you to balance your time between things that you have to do, for example work, studying, or managing your home, with pleasurable activities such as seeing friends and having time on your own to relax.

Important Facts to Consider When Planning an Activity Program

- Try to include a few short breaks each day in your busy schedule. Even if you are working in a demanding job or looking after young children, it should be possible to ensure that you have at least a 15-minute break in the morning and afternoon, as well as a lunch break of at least half an hour.
- Do *not* be tempted to carry out long periods of activities without breaks, even if you feel that you have a lot of energy. You are likely to pay for it later and then *feel* that you need to rest for a long time to feel better.

- Do *not* be tempted to catch up with rest at the weekend. Once you start taking regular breaks in the day, you should feel less tired at the weekend and have a bit more energy. Try to plan a few 'pleasurable' activities for the weekend, as well as a bit of time to catch up with chores, and so on, if necessary.

Refer to your target breakdown sheet on pages 56–8 for guidance on some of the activities that you may like to include in your activity program.

Steps to Creating an Activity Program

Planning Activities

- Write a list of activities that you would like to do during the next week on your activity program. (A blank activity program can be found on page 82.) For each activity, specify how often you want to do it and how long you want to spend on it on each occasion; e.g. 'Leave work by 5 p.m. two days a week'; 'Meet a friend once a week for one hour'.
- Use your activity diaries for guidance on the total amount of time to be spent on each activity during the week.
- When writing your first activity program, aim for about as much 'overall' activity as you are having at present. So, for example, if you do all of your chores at the weekend, break up the amount of time that you usually spend on them into small chunks to do on two or three days.
- Remember to make your activity times manageable chunks, rather than one long session; e.g. if you plan to do some gardening at a weekend, plan two half-hour periods rather than a solid hour.

Planning Relaxation Time

Whether you are working, studying, or managing a home and/or looking after children, regular time for relaxation is important. Taking breaks can help you to feel a lot better and is likely to contribute to your having a bit more energy to do the things that you want to do in the evenings and at weekends. What you find relaxing is a very personal thing. It may be reading a book, listening to music, gardening, or taking a long bath.

In order to plan relaxation time:

- Look at the activity diaries that you have completed during the previous fortnight and estimate the amount of rest or relaxation time you have had. (You may find that on some days you rested very little, but at weekends you rested for much of the time.)
- Divide the total amount of rest you have taken during the day in the past two weeks by 14 to calculate the amount of relaxation time to be taken each day. (This will mean increasing rests on some days and reducing them on others.)
- Write down on your activity program the number of breaks to be taken each day, and the length of each one. If you are working or studying, you will need to consider what is achievable in relation to your commitments. For example, you might take two 15-minute breaks and one one-hour break each day; or you might take three half-hour breaks each day.

Examples of an Initial Activity Program

For someone who works full-time:
- To have at least two 15-minute breaks and a half-hour lunch break every day.
- To leave work on time at least twice a week.
- To have half an hour of exercise at least twice a week.
- To spend one hour daily doing something relaxing; e.g. listening to music, watching television.
- To go out socially once a week for two hours.
- To go to bed by 11.00 p.m. every day during the week.

For someone who cares for family/home all of the time:
- To have one 15-minute break at home in the morning and one in the afternoon every day.
- To have a half-hour break at lunch time every day.
- To spend one hour, twice a day, cleaning/cooking/doing other chores.
- To go for two 15-minute walks every day.
- To go out with friends and/or partner every week for two hours.
- To stop chores by 9.00 p.m. every day.
- To spend at least one hour a day on a hobby or reading.

Recording Your Activities

You will already be used to recording your activities in your activity diary. It is important that you continue to write down details of what you are doing for each hour of the day in your activity diary once you have begun your activity program so that you can monitor your progress.

What to Expect When You Start Your Activity Program

It may take a few weeks for you to start feeling better. Initially, when you begin your activity program you may find that your fatigue and other symptoms remain the same or slightly increase. This is particularly likely to happen if you significantly change your usual routine or start a new activity. On the other hand, if you are introducing more regular breaks into your day, you may notice a slight decrease in your fatigue.

Even if you notice a slight increase in your symptoms, it is important that you maintain your activity program as far as possible. Your symptoms should gradually decrease after a few weeks.

Changing Your Activity Levels

Once you have established a more consistent pattern of activity and rest, you will be in a position to start *gradually* to introduce new activities; for example, hobbies or social events. This will probably be two weeks or so after you start your program, when you are more used to doing things at regular times.

- Look at the activity program that you made yourself for the past week, and ask yourself, for each different activity: 'How successful was I at completing it?' You may find it helpful to refer to Table 7.1 on page 74 for guidance.

When Should I Introduce New Activities?

- *When the overall success of the previous activity program reaches about 75 per cent.* It is important that you feel that you are managing your program reasonably well before adding in new activities. Otherwise you may end up feeling a little out of control. It is just as important to consider your success in achieving regular time for relaxation as it is to consider whether or not you have done your planned exercise.
- *When you have achieved a target.* When you have achieved a particular target, you may find that you have the time to introduce another activity; e.g. if you have completed a course at college, you may plan to do another. Or, if you have achieved a target of leaving work on time twice a week, you may consider leaving work on time every day. Alternatively, you may start working on a new target; e.g. meeting up with friends regularly.
- *If, for reasons beyond your control, you are unable to continue a particular target.* Sometimes you will find that you plan targets that are not manageable for a variety of reasons. So, for example, if one of your targets was to go to a yoga class once a week, but the class was cancelled because not enough people enrolled, then you may decide to join a Pilates class or practise yoga exercises at home until the class reopens.
- It is *not* necessary for your fatigue to have decreased for you to increase or start a new activity.

81

Activity program

1 _____
2 _____
3 _____
4 _____
5 _____
6 _____
7 _____
8 _____
9 _____
10 _____
11 _____
12 _____
13 _____
14 _____
15 _____
16 _____
17 _____
18 _____
19 _____
20 _____

How often should I review my program?

Reviewing your program each week will help you to assess your progress, even though you may make changes to it only, say, once a fortnight, or once a month. From now on, set aside 15–30 minutes a week to review your homework and to plan your next activity program.

Remember to make time for relaxation, with no specific activity allocated.

Keeping a Target Achievement Record

When you feel that you have established a good routine and are *consistently* maintaining your activity program, you may feel that your activity and sleep diaries are no longer necessary or helpful. If this is the case, then you may like to record your activities on a target achievement record instead. This record will help you track your progress, but requires you only to make a tick in a box, rather than actually writing details of what you have done.

Target achievement records are less time-consuming than activity diaries, but they still need to be completed accurately. If you do not record sufficient information, it will become difficult for you to track your progress or decide how to change your activity program. So it is important that you are not tempted to use these records until you feel confident about your routine.

An example of a completed target achievement record, and a blank record sheet for you to photocopy, are included on pages 84–5.

What Do I Have To Do?

- Write down the contents of your activity program on the left-hand side of your target achievement record; e.g. get up by 8 a.m., read a newspaper for 15 minutes daily, etc.
- Tick the appropriate boxes as you complete these activities throughout the day, so that you can easily monitor your progress.
- For targets that you do not attempt, put an X in the appropriate box.
- For targets that you attempt, but do not manage to carry on for the planned time, record how long you did manage; e.g. against 'Go for a half-hour walk' you might note '20 minutes'.
- If you start using the target achievement records and find after a week or so that you do not find them helpful, then return to using activity diaries.

Sample completed target achievement record

Fortnight beginning ....

Target	Mon	Tue	Wed	Thu	Fri	Sat	Sun	Mon	Tue	Wed	Thu	Fri	Sat	Sun
To get up by 8 a.m.	✓	8.20	✓	✓	✓	9.00	8.45	✓	✓	✓	✓	8.15	9.30	9.10
To walk for ½ hour × 2 daily	✓ ✗	✓✓	20 mins	✓✓	✓✓	✓ ✗	✗ ✓	✓✓	✓✓	15 mins	✓✓	✓✓	✗ 45 mins	✓✓
To read for ½ hour × 2 daily	✓✓	✓✓	✗ ✓	✓✓	✓✓	✗	✓ ✗	✓✓	✓✓	✓✓	✓✓	40 mins	✗ ✗	✓✓
To have an hour's rest in chair at 10 a.m.	✓	✓	✓	✓	½ hrs	1¼ hrs	✓	✓	✓	✓	✓	45 mins	✗	✓
To do chores for ½ hour × 2 daily	✓✓	✓✓	✓ ✗	✓✓	✓✓	10 mins ✓	✓ ✗	✓✓	✓✓	✓✓	✓✓	✓✓	✗ ✗	✗ ✓✓
To have an hour's rest in chair at 1 p.m.	✓	✓	1¼ hrs	✓	✓	2 hrs	✓	✓	✓	✓	½ hrs	✓	✓	✓
To meet a friend for coffee × 2 weekly for 1 hour		✓			✓			✓			Met for lunch			
To swim × 2 weekly for 20 minutes			✓			✓				✓				✓
To have an hour's rest in chair at 4 p.m.	✓	✓	✓	✓	✓	✓	✓	✓	✓	✓	1½ hrs	45 mins	✗	✓
To prepare evening meal × 3 weekly for family	✓			✓		✓			✓			✓		✓
Enquire about voluntary work		✓ online												
Comments					late night	felt v. ill	better day			enjoyed swim				

84

Target achievement record

Target	Mon	Tue	Wed	Thu	Fri	Sat	Sun	Mon	Tue	Wed	Thu	Fri	Sat	Sun

8

Overcoming Unhelpful Thinking Patterns

For the past few weeks or months you will have been working on establishing a regular pattern of activity, rest and sleep. We hope that by now you feel that you are making some progress, feeling a little less fatigued and experiencing fewer symptoms. However, sometimes progress can seem very slow, and there may be times when you feel despondent and that it is a real struggle to carry out your activity program.

This chapter aims to help you to understand a little more about how unhelpful thoughts and beliefs can hamper your progress and how to stop this happening. We have divided this chapter into two sections:

- In Section 1, we discuss how all our lives are influenced by the way we think about things. We then describe common unhelpful thoughts reported by people with CFS. Finally, we discuss ways of identifying and challenging unhelpful thoughts.
- In Section 2, we set about helping you to tackle deeper unhelpful beliefs. This section will be particularly relevant if you have a number of unhelpful thoughts that appear to be related to a particular theme. It may also be helpful if you find that, even if you challenge your unhelpful thoughts frequently, they keep coming back.

When Would Be a Good Time to Start Working Through This Chapter?

We would suggest that you start working through this chapter when you feel reasonably confident about managing a consistent pattern of activity and rest. This may be a few weeks or a few months after writing your first activity program.

SECTION 1: TACKLING UNHELPFUL THOUGHTS

Our lives are influenced by five interconnected areas:

- thoughts (beliefs, images, memories);
- feelings (moods or emotions);
- behaviors (what we do; e.g. activity, sleep, rest);
- physical reactions (fatigue, pain, dizziness, changes in energy levels, sleep, appetite, etc.);
- environment (what happens in our life, both past and present).

Each area directly influences each of the other four areas, as shown in Figure 8.1 on page 88. Understanding this interaction may help you to understand and manage certain problems more effectively.

For example:

- If someone gives you a present (behavior) it is likely that you would feel happy (emotion).
- If you cut your finger (behavior), it is likely that you would feel pain (physical reaction) and, depending on how bad the cut is, you may feel dizzy or sick (physical reactions) and feel cross with yourself for being careless (emotions).
- If you pass an exam/receive promotion (environment), you are likely to have positive thoughts about yourself (thoughts) and be happy (emotion), and may go out and celebrate (behavior).

You can *think* about a situation in a variety of ways. The way that you *think* about the situation will determine how you *feel*.

87

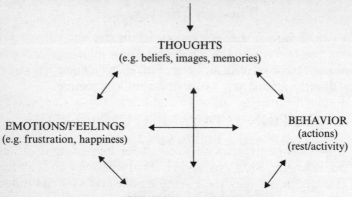

ENVIRONMENT/LIFE CHANGES/SITUATIONS

THOUGHTS
(e.g. beliefs, images, memories)

EMOTIONS/FEELINGS
(e.g. frustration, happiness)

BEHAVIOR
(actions)
(rest/activity)

PHYSICAL REACTIONS
(symptoms – e.g. pain, fatigue, dizziness,
changes in sleep, appetite, energy levels)

Figure 8.1   How aspects of our lives interconnect

Example:
It is 8.00 p.m., and your guests should have been at your house for dinner half an hour ago.

Possible thoughts	*Possible feelings*
• They're caught up in traffic and will be here soon.	content
• Thank goodness they're late. It has given me some extra time to get myself and the food ready.	relieved
• Maybe they're not coming and just couldn't be bothered to phone	irritated
• They've probably just forgotten. I'll give them a couple of minutes and then phone them.	understanding
• They obviously don't like me any more, otherwise they would have been here on time.	sad

You can see that each different thought is likely to lead to a different feeling or emotion; e.g. relief, sadness, irritation. It is likely that, as a result of these thoughts and feelings, people would behave in different ways. For example:

- the 'content' person may have been 'relaxed' if/when the guests arrived and had an 'enjoyable' evening;
- the 'irritated' person may have been 'curt' to their guests and had a 'difficult' evening.

If we change the way we think about something it can affect our behavior, emotions, and physical reactions, and can lead to changes in our lifestyle. Changing our behavior can influence the way we feel both physically and emotionally.

So, using the example above, if the 'irritated' person changed their thoughts to 'They're probably just caught up in traffic and will be here soon', they are likely to feel more 'relaxed' when their guests arrive and, as a consequence, have a pleasant evening.

Changes in our life will influence our emotions, physical feelings, thoughts, and behavior. It is likely that promotion, passing exams, winning the lottery, and so on will make us feel happy, feel good about ourselves, and inclined to celebrate. Failing exams, illness, relationship break-ups, and financial difficulties are changes in our lives that may make us feel upset, worried, stressed, and tired, and may lead us to feel down, withdraw from others, and so on.

Unhelpful Thoughts Associated with CFS

If you are suffering from a debilitating illness such as chronic fatigue syndrome, it may be difficult at times to retain a positive attitude when you feel so unwell, your life has become restricted, and your future appears uncertain. At times you may feel frustrated, demoralized, or worried about your health and associated problems. These feelings can make it harder for you to make progress in overcoming your illness.

When you begin your activity program, you may have thoughts such as:

- 'I am feeling more fatigued than when I started the program! What's the point in continuing?'
- 'I haven't managed to get up at the agreed time for the last few days, it's just too hard!'

These are examples of 'unhelpful thoughts' which may make it difficult at times for you to continue with your activity program.

We have noticed that many people with CFS have unhelpful thoughts that can be divided into two main areas:

- fears about their illness;
- extremely high personal standards and self-expectations.

Fears about the Illness

These thoughts are quite understandable, as the symptoms of chronic fatigue syndrome are both debilitating and distressing, and 'experts', relatives, and friends alike have differing attitudes not only about the illness itself, but also about what you should and shouldn't do.

Here is an example of how an unhelpful thought related to fears about illness affected other areas of a person's life:

Situation	Woke up feeling exhausted and very achy after walking too far the previous day.
Thought	'I must be getting worse.'
Behavior	Rested for most of the day.
Emotions	*Worried* about making CFS worse. *Annoyed* for giving in to tiredness.
Physical reaction	Worsening/more awareness of physical symptoms; e.g. fatigue and aching muscles.

Can you think of any personal examples of how thoughts about CFS have influenced other aspects of your life? If so, please write them in the spaces provided on the next page.

Situation

Thought

Behavior

Emotion

Physical reaction

Having Extremely High Personal Standards and Self-Expectations

Many people with CFS say that before they developed the illness they were very busy, energetic people: 'driven', successful, with high expectations of themselves (in other words, perfectionists). The effects of CFS can make it very difficult to maintain previous personal standards or activity levels, and this can lead to:

- being overly self-critical;
- worrying about starting new things, fearing not being able to do them well enough;
- doubting your own judgment, making it hard to complete tasks;
- focusing on things that you *haven't* done;
- feeling guilty about relaxing when you haven't completed a task;
- feeling frustrated about doing so much less than you used to be able to do.

Here is an example of how unhelpful thoughts related to perfectionism affected a person with CFS:

Situation	Didn't achieve all that I planned to do today.
Thought	I'm useless! I should have handed in the essay by now.
Emotions	*Frustrated* about not completing the tasks that I set myself.

	Worried about missing another deadline.
Behavior	Unable to relax or concentrate on any one thing.
Physical reaction	Feeling more fatigued.

Can you think of any personal examples of how 'perfectionist' thoughts have influenced other aspects of your life since you developed CFS? If so, please write them in the spaces provided below.

Situation

Thought

Behavior

Emotion

Physical reaction

As well as the unhelpful thoughts mentioned above, you might from time to time have unhelpful thoughts about a variety of things related or unrelated to your CFS; for example, relationship issues, finances, moving house. These thoughts may also make you feel a bit upset or low in mood, and may in turn negatively affect your thoughts about your CFS.

Characteristics of Unhelpful Thoughts

Unhelpful thoughts are:

- *automatic*: as with all thoughts, unhelpful ones tend to pop into our head rapidly and unexpectedly, without any deliberate or conscious effort;
- *distorted*: they are usually not entirely accurate;
- *plausible*: we accept them as facts, and do not question them;
- *persistent*: they can be difficult to switch off;
- *durable*: it can be useful to view unhelpful thoughts as prejudices as they can be hard to change.

How Do I Identify and Record
My Unhelpful Thoughts?

Try to notice what goes through your mind when you have a strong feeling, a strong reaction to something, or a change in your mood.

Write down your unhelpful thoughts as soon as possible so that you remember the details. A good way to do this is to use an 'unhelpful thoughts diary' with headings like the one below. A blank diary can be found on page 96.

Date	Situation	Emotion	Unhelpful thoughts
	What was I doing at the time of the thoughts?	How did I feel? Rate intensity (0–100%)	What thoughts went through my mind just before I started to feel this way? Rate belief in each thought (0–100%)

- In the 'Situation' column, write down what you were doing or thinking about just before having a strong feeling or change in your emotion/mood.
- In the 'Emotion' column, write down the emotion or feeling that you had when you had the unhelpful thought(s). Then write down the intensity of your emotion on a 0–100% scale.
- In the 'Unhelpful thoughts' column, write down the actual thought that went through your mind. If you have more

than one unhelpful thought connected with the situation, either

(a) draw a line under the thought that you feel particularly provokes the emotion, or
(b) break down your thoughts into separate ones and write a diary entry for each.

- Underneath, in the same column, write down how much you believe each thought, on a 0–100% scale, where 0% means that you do not believe it at all and 100% means that you believe the thought completely, without any doubts.

Initially it can be difficult to detect your 'unhelpful' thoughts. After all, we are not used to focusing on what we are thinking about!

Sometimes people feel a bit uncertain about writing down their unhelpful thoughts, but look at it as the first step to overcoming them.

An example of a completed unhelpful thoughts diary may be found on the next page. A blank unhelpful thoughts diary may be found on page 96.

For How Long Should I Complete My Unhelpful Thoughts Diary?

It is a good idea to write down your thoughts in your unhelpful thoughts diary for a few days, or until you feel that you can clearly distinguish between a *thought* and a *feeling* (emotion). This can be a little tricky at first, so it is worth spending a bit of time on it to make sure that you know the difference between thoughts and emotions, before moving on.

Example of a completed unhelpful thoughts diary

Date	Situation	Emotion	Unhelpful thoughts
	What was I doing at the time of the thoughts?	How did I feel? Rate intensity (0–100%)	What thoughts went through my mind just before I started to feel this way? Rate belief in each thought (0–100%)
1 Feb.	Sitting down after a ten-minute walk feeling exhausted.	Frustrated 70% Worried 80%	I feel so tired, *I must be making myself worse. I am now too tired to do anything. 80%
3 Feb.	Meeting up with old friends from work.	Sad 80%	**I feel so out of touch with everyone.
			**I haven't worked for over a year and have nothing to contribute to the conversation.
			**They must think that I am very boring.

*Thought that particularly provoked emotion is underlined.
**Thought is broken down into separate thoughts.

Use the blank chart on the next page to record any unhelpful thoughts you have had recently, using the example above for guidance.

Unhelpful thoughts diary

Date	Situation	Emotion	Unhelpful thoughts
	What was I doing at the time of the thoughts?	How did I feel? Rate intensity (0–100%)	What thoughts went through my mind just before I started to feel this way? Rate belief in each thought (0–100%)

Standing Back from Your Unhelpful Thoughts

Once you have identified some unhelpful thoughts, the very act of taking a step back from them can in itself be very powerful, enabling you to see them for what they really are: not facts, just thoughts. Prefixing an unhelpful thought with 'I am having the thought that . . .' can help you to achieve this aim.

Although some people find that standing back from their thoughts can lead to a positive change in the way they feel, this is not always the case. The next section shows how you can identify thinking errors by dissecting each unhelpful thought, and discusses ways of challenging your unhelpful thoughts, helping you to look at things in a more balanced way.

Challenging Unhelpful Thoughts

Once you have identified some unhelpful thoughts and have written them down, then the next step is to challenge them.

Why Is It Important to Challenge Unhelpful Thoughts?

We have already discussed how the way we *think* about something will determine how we *feel*, and how the way we *feel* will often determine what we *do*. Unhelpful thoughts can affect how we feel and what we do in a negative way. Challenging these thoughts will help you to look at things in a more positive and helpful way, which will directly benefit the way you feel, and may lead to more positive behavior.

When you start to challenge your unhelpful thoughts, we suggest that you look back at the unhelpful thoughts diaries that you have completed and pick just one thought that you would like to challenge, following the three steps outlined below. When you have managed to challenge one unhelpful thought, you can either challenge another that you have already written down on your unhelpful thoughts diary, or wait until you have another unhelpful thought and then challenge that one.

The 'new thoughts diary' expands on the unhelpful thoughts

diary, adding three new stages:

1 *Evaluate your thoughts* to look for unhelpful thinking patterns.
2 *Suggest alternative thoughts* that are more realistic or helpful.
3 *Think of an action plan* to provide yourself with practical strategies to help you to break old habits of thinking and strengthen new ones.

Completing a new thoughts diary on this model will help you to monitor your progress in challenging your unhelpful thoughts. Detailed instructions on how to do this, with completed examples and a blank for you to photocopy, are to be found on pages 103–8.

When you start to challenge your unhelpful thoughts using your new thoughts diary, you can stop completing your unhelpful thoughts diary.

Step 1: Evaluate Your Unhelpful Thoughts

Evaluating your thoughts involves detecting *thinking errors*: these are unhelpful thinking patterns that seem plausible, but often involve distortions of reality. This process will help you to stand back and dissect your thoughts rather than accepting them as facts.

• Look at the examples of unhelpful thinking patterns on the next page.
• Look back at some of the unhelpful thoughts that you have written down. Can you identify any thinking errors?

When you start to evaluate your thoughts, you may notice that you have a tendency towards one or two thinking errors in particular.

When you have been able to detect some thinking errors in a few of your unhelpful thoughts, move on to step 2.

Unhelpful patterns of thinking

Unhelpful thinking pattern (thinking error/distortion)	Description	Example
All-or-nothing thinking, also called black-and-white thinking	Looking at a situation as two extremes only, instead of a continuum.	'If I can't stay out until late, then there is no point in going out at all.'
Overgeneralization	Making a negative assumption that because something has happened once, it will naturally happen again.	'I felt much worse when I increased my exercise before, so I am bound to feel the same the next time I increase my exercise.'
Eliminating the positive	Dwelling on bad experiences and discounting positive aspects.	'I have had a terrible week and I have achieved nothing.'
'Should' and 'must' statements	Fixed expectations of how you think you or others should behave. You may overestimate how bad it is if these expectations are not met.	'I should be able to cope better by now; I'm not trying hard enough.' 'I must make more of an effort in future.'
Catastrophizing	Getting things out of proportion, so that they appear worse than they really are.	'My muscles ache and I feel more tired today. I must be doing some permanent damage to myself.'
Emotional reasoning	Taking a feeling as being evidence of fact. You 'feel' (believe) it so strongly that you discount evidence to the contrary.	'I *feel* a real failure; I am no better now than I was a few months ago.'
Labelling	Putting a 'fixed' or 'global' label on yourself or others without considering evidence that doesn't support it.	'I'm incompetent.' 'My colleagues are totally insensitive.'
Mental filter	Paying undue attention to one negative detail instead of seeing the whole picture.	'One or two of my exam marks were dreadful (even though others were good); I don't deserve to pass my degree.'
Mind-reading	Believing that you know what others are thinking, without considering other more likely possibilities.	'They think that just because I don't look ill, I am not ill.'
Personalization	Believing that others are behaving in a certain (negative) way because of you.	'My doctor was irritable because I went to see him for two weeks running.'
Tunnel vision	Seeing only the negative aspects of a situation.	'I feel just as tired as I did three months ago; there has been no improvement in my illness.'

Step 2: Suggesting Alternative Thoughts That Are More Helpful and Realistic

The following questions aim to help you to look for more helpful and realistic alternatives to your unhelpful thoughts by:

- looking at the situation from another point of view;
- finding evidence that does not support them.

Choose one unhelpful thought and go through questions 1–10 with it. Write your answers down.

1 Have I had experiences that indicate that this thought is not true all of the time?
2 Am I assuming that this view is the only one, whereas another person might look at the same thing in a different way?
3 If my best friend or someone I loved had been in a similar situation, would I say the things that I have said to myself to him or to her? What might I say to them?
4 If my best friend or someone that is close to me knew that I was thinking these things, what would they say to me?
5 What is the actual evidence that this thought is true?
6 Is there any evidence that this thought may not be entirely accurate?
7 Are there any small things that contradict my thoughts that I might be discounting as not important?
8 Am I blaming myself for something that wasn't entirely my fault?
9 Am I being too self-critical and expecting too much of myself?
10 What are the advantages and disadvantages of thinking this way?

After writing down your answers to the above questions, consider alternative thoughts. These should be more balanced and helpful than those that you have written in the 'Unhelpful thoughts' column of your unhelpful thoughts diary. One or two of your alternative thoughts may be the same as answers that you have written to questions 1–10.

Step 3: Writing an Action Plan

Detecting thinking errors and suggesting alternative thoughts may not always be enough to help you to feel better or to convince you that your thoughts are distorted or incorrect. Writing an action plan will provide you with practical strategies to help you to break old habits of thinking and strengthen new ones. In some instances, having an action plan may help you to build up evidence that contradicts your unhelpful thoughts.

The type of action plan that you make will depend on your unhelpful thoughts. Below are some ideas for action plans that may be helpful for different kinds of unhelpful thoughts.

Thoughts about not making much progress:
• Write down improvements that you have made, however small.
• Reread relevant chapters from this book to see if there is anything else that you can do to further your improvement.

Thoughts about the symptoms getting worse:
• Reread the relevant chapters from this book.
• If you have new and severe symptoms that last for more than a few days, speak to your doctor.

Thoughts related to not achieving what you want to achieve/doing things well, etc. (perfectionism):
• If you are focusing on a particular negative aspect of yourself or your situation (e.g. if you feel responsible for something that has not gone well), construct a 'responsibility pie chart'. See page 102 for an example.
• Write a list of things that you have achieved, however small.

Thoughts about not managing to do day-to-day activities:
• Allocate a few minutes a day to doing something that you are putting off or finding difficult.

Thoughts related to doing something new:
• Allocate a time to buy materials for a new hobby; e.g. painting.

- Allocate time each day to prepare for a course, plan how to get there, etc.
- Speak to prospective employers/tutors/course leaders/voluntary work leaders, and so on, about your concerns.

Thoughts about loneliness:
- Contact friends again or explore ways of making new friends.

Thoughts about never having time for yourself:
- Prioritize 'quality' time for yourself each day.

Constructing a 'Responsibility Pie Chart'

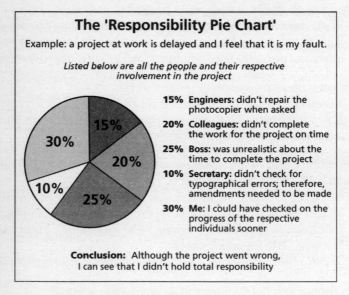

The 'Responsibility Pie Chart'

Example: a project at work is delayed and I feel that it is my fault.

Listed below are all the people and their respective involvement in the project

15% Engineers: didn't repair the photocopier when asked

20% Colleagues: didn't complete the work for the project on time

25% Boss: was unrealistic about the time to complete the project

10% Secretary: didn't check for typographical errors; therefore, amendments needed to be made

30% Me: I could have checked on the progress of the respective individuals sooner

Conclusion: Although the project went wrong, I can see that I didn't hold total responsibility

Figure 8.2   The 'Responsibility Pie Chart'

If you are focusing on a negative aspect of either yourself or a situation, it can be helpful to think about all the other factors, apart from that particular aspect, that may be involved. For example, if you feel responsible or blamed for something, it can be worth thinking about the other factors or people that may have affected the outcome.

Make a list of them; then draw a circle and allocate them percentages according to how much responsibility you think each has for the outcome/situation, leaving yourself until last (see Figure 8.2 on the previous page). You will probably find that you end up with a picture in which you take a much less prominent part than you originally thought.

How to Complete Your New Thoughts Diary

Using the steps outlined on the last few pages, you can begin to keep a new thoughts diary to help you identify and overcome your unhelpful thoughts. Two examples of completed diary entries are shown on pages 106–7, and there is a blank form for you to photocopy on page 108.

The first four columns of the new thoughts diary are the same as your unhelpful thoughts diary.

- Date: record the date to help you keep track of your progress.
- In the 'Situation' column, write down what you were doing or thinking about prior to having a strong feeling or change in your mood.
- In the 'Emotion' column, write down the emotion or feeling that you had at the time that you had your unhelpful thought. Rate how strong your emotion was on a 0–100% scale.
- In the 'Unhelpful thoughts' column, write down the actual thought(s) that went through your mind. Rate how much you believe each thought, on a 0–100% scale.

In the next four columns you record the steps of your challenge to the unhelpful thought:

- In the 'Evidence for and against your thoughts' column, first write down any thinking errors that are apparent in your unhelpful thoughts; then write down your answers to questions 1–10 on page 100. Not all of the questions will be relevant, but try to answer at least three or four.

- In the 'Alternative thoughts' column, write down two or three alternative thoughts after reflecting on the information that you have written in the previous column. The idea is for these thoughts to be more balanced and helpful. Rate each new thought in terms of how much you believe it on a 0–100% scale.

- In the 'Outcome' column, rerate your belief in your unhelpful thoughts, and the intensity of your emotions, each on a 0–100% scale. Re-rating your beliefs and emotions in this way will indicate how helpful your alternative thoughts are. If there is no change in your ratings of emotions and belief in your unhelpful thought after you have come up with alternative thoughts, you may like to try to think of more alternatives, or come back to it later.

- In the 'Action plan' column, write down any strategies you can think of that will help you to overcome your unhelpful thinking patterns, improve your situation, help you to feel better, etc. Depending on what you come up with, it may be helpful to include time in your activity program to carry out your action plan.

Points to Bear In Mind When Tackling Unhelpful Thoughts

- Do not give up if you find the procedure difficult at first. Constantly evaluating and challenging our thoughts is not something that we normally do, so many people do not find it easy. Follow the guidelines carefully and in time you are likely to find it easier and see how it can help you.

- It can be difficult to think of 'evidence against your unhelpful thoughts' or 'alternative thoughts' when you feel upset, angry, etc. However, it is important that you write down your unhelpful thoughts as soon as you can, so that you do not forget any details. If you are unable to think of evidence against your unhelpful thoughts or alternative ones straight away, do not worry: do something else until you feel calmer; and then you will be in a better position to tackle them.

- Alternative thoughts are ones that help you to change the way you feel about a situation or problem. They do not have to be relentlessly positive!
- It will take time and practice to build up belief in your alternative responses.
- Try not to feel discouraged if you find the same type of thought recurring; this is likely to happen if unhelpful thinking is well established. Keep challenging your thought however often it occurs; this will help to reduce your belief in the original thought.
- Eventually, you may be able to challenge your unhelpful thoughts in your head. Initially, however, writing them down is easier, and will help you to be more objective.
- Remember that there is no right or wrong way of thinking. The aim of challenging your unhelpful thoughts is to help you to feel better.

New thoughts diary, example 1

Date	Situation	Emotion	Unhelpful thoughts	Evidence for and against your thoughts	Alternative thoughts	Outcome	Action plan
	What was I doing at the time of my thoughts?	How did I feel? Rate intensity (0–100%)	What thoughts went through my mind just before I started to feel this way? Rate belief (0–100%)	Note down thinking errors (see page 99) Write answers to the questions on page 100	Write alternative thoughts after answering questions in previous column. Rate belief in each thought (0–100%)	Re-rate belief in thought and intensity of emotion (0–100%)	What can I do now?
1 Jan.	Watching TV, thinking about what I had done during the day	Frustrated (80%)	I have had an awful day, I don't seem to have achieved anything (95%)	Eliminating the positive 2 Others may say that I had managed to get up and get dressed and had done a few jobs 3 No, I wouldn't say these things to my best friend if she were in a similar situation. I would tell her that she'd done well under the circumstances 5 No evidence I have done something today	Although I have not done all I planned for the day, I have done about half. (90%) A few weeks ago, if I had felt as I did today, I would probably have stayed in bed all day 90%	Unhelpful thought (40%) Emotion (40%)	Praise myself for what I have achieved, rather than focusing on what I haven't done Start afresh tomorrow Write a list of things that I achieve each day

New thoughts diary, example 2

Date	Situation	Emotion	Unhelpful thoughts	Evidence for and against your thoughts	Alternative thoughts	Outcome	Action plan
	What was I doing at the time of my thoughts?	How did I feel? Rate intensity (0–100%)	What thoughts went through my mind just before I started to feel this way? Rate belief (0–100%)	Note down thinking errors (see page 99) Write answers to the questions on page 100	Write alternative thoughts after answering questions in previous column. Rate belief in each thought (0–100%)	Rerate belief in thought and intensity of emotion (0–100%)	What can I do now?
2 Jan.	Feeling ill, woke up with swollen glands	Fed up (100%)	This is never-ending (100%)	Catastrophizing; overgeneralizing 1 Yes, I don't always feel like this 2 Another person may say that my swollen glands are only temporary 5 I have no evidence that this thought is true 7 Maybe I am forgetting that there are times when I am feeling better	I am actually much better than I was a few months ago despite having swollen glands today (100%) Maybe my swollen glands are an indication that I have been doing too much lately and need to calm down a bit (80%)	Thought (65%) Emotion (60%)	Stick to my program as much as possible

New thoughts diary

Date	Situation	Emotion	Unhelpful thoughts	Evidence for and against your thoughts	Alternative thoughts	Outcome	Action plan
	What was I doing at the time of my thoughts?	How did I feel? Rate intensity (0–100%)	What thoughts went through my mind just before I started to feel this way? Rate belief (0–100%)	Note down thinking errors (see page 99) Write answers to the questions on page 100	Write alternative thoughts after answering questions in previous column. Rate belief in each thought (0–100%)	Re-rate belief in thought and intensity of emotion (0–100%)	What can I do now?

SECTION 2: TACKLING UNHELPFUL ASSUMPTIONS AND CORE BELIEFS

Addressing your unhelpful thoughts as described in Section 1 of this chapter may be all that is necessary to help you to overcome or deal with certain problems more effectively. However, if you find that you have several such thoughts based on a single theme, or thoughts that come up again and again however much you challenge them, you may find this section helpful.

When Should I Move On to This Section?

We would suggest that you start working through this section only when you feel confident in challenging unhelpful thoughts.

The Different Levels of Belief

We all have different levels of belief. For our purposes here it is useful to identify three, working from those nearest to the surface down to the deepest.

Automatic Thoughts

Automatic thoughts are the most accessible level, and after some practice are fairly easy to identify. These are generally the things that we say to ourselves. They can be a direct reflection of our assumptions or core beliefs (for examples of these, see below) or they may be driven by them; for example, a thought such as 'I didn't do well in my exam' may be driven by a core belief 'I am not good enough', a thought such as 'I don't have any friends' may come from a belief that 'I am not lovable'. You have already worked on your unhelpful automatic thoughts in the previous section of this chapter.

Assumptions

These operate as rules that guide our daily actions and expectations. They are less obvious than automatic thoughts. They usually take the form of 'should' statements, or 'if . . . then . . .' sentences. Examples are:

'I should be better by now'
'I should be back at work by now'
'If I don't get at least 75 per cent in my exam, then I'm incompetent'
'If I'm not talkative when I go out, then people will think I'm boring'
'If I ask for help, then people will think that I am weak'

The development of assumptions is influenced by our core beliefs.

Core Beliefs

These are our deepest level of belief. Core beliefs are absolute statements that we may hold about ourselves, other people, or the world. Examples are:

'I am unlovable'   'I am loveable'
'I am a failure'   'I am good enough'
'Other people are   'I am as good as other people'
better than me'

Where Do Assumptions and Core Beliefs Come From?

On the basis of experiences that we have while growing up, we form conclusions (beliefs or assumptions) in order to try to make sense of ourselves, other people, and the world. If we encounter traumatic experiences – for example, bullying, abuse, or excessive criticism – we are likely to develop negative or unhelpful core beliefs or assumptions.

Later in life, these beliefs or assumptions may be activated in certain situations, resulting in our thinking, feeling, and behaving in ways that may further exacerbate unhelpful thoughts and feelings. (Please see Figure 8.3 on the next page for a diagram showing how this can work.)

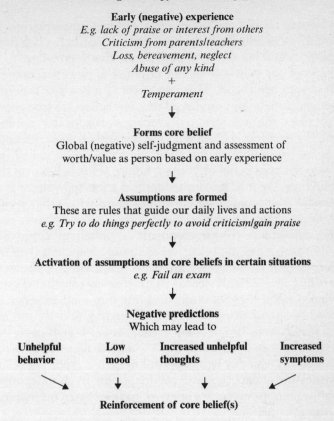

Early (negative) experience
E.g. lack of praise or interest from others
Criticism from parents/teachers
Loss, bereavement, neglect
Abuse of any kind
+
Temperament
↓

Forms core belief
Global (negative) self-judgment and assessment of
worth/value as person based on early experience
↓

Assumptions are formed
These are rules that guide our daily lives and actions
e.g. Try to do things perfectly to avoid criticism/gain praise
↓

Activation of assumptions and core beliefs in certain situations
e.g. Fail an exam
↓

Negative predictions
Which may lead to

| **Unhelpful behavior** | **Low mood** | **Increased unhelpful thoughts** | **Increased symptoms** |

Reinforcement of core belief(s)

Figure 8.3   The formation of (negative) core beliefs and possible consequences

The rules and beliefs that we acquire as young children are not necessarily true, but we take them as such as we are unable to be flexible in our thinking until we are older. For example, if a young child is scratched or bitten by a cat, they may think that all cats are malicious and be frightened of them. It is unlikely that they will change their attitude about them until they are older; then, when they see friends playing with cats, they may learn that some cats are friendly, and some cats are not. When we get older, not only do we learn to be more flexible in our rules and beliefs, we

111

also learn to change our behavior according to the situation. For example, we usually learn that it is safe to approach a dog that is wagging its tail, but not to approach one that is growling.

Some of our beliefs from our childhood, however, may stay with us into adulthood. This can occur as a result of traumatic experiences, or being convinced that our beliefs are true even as we get older, through repeatedly facing situations that reinforce them. For example, a child who is constantly being criticized at home and at school might conclude that he/she is bad, and develop the core belief of being a failure. This belief may then be reinforced later in life; for example if a job application is not successful. Persistent negative interactions with other people, such as observing a highly successful sibling who receives much praise, can lead to the development of 'unhelpful' core beliefs about others; for example 'others are more competent than me'.

Because our core beliefs help us to make sense of the world at a young age, it rarely occurs to us to assess whether they are the most useful ways of understanding our adult experiences. Instead, we tend to go on acting, thinking, and feeling as if these beliefs were 100 per cent true. Also, although many core beliefs stem from childhood, we can acquire new negative core beliefs at any age, through powerful negative experiences such as witnessing or experiencing trauma; living in chaotic, unpredictable circumstances; or experiencing persistent unhappiness for whatever reason.

What Is the Point of Trying to Change Assumptions and Core Beliefs?

Learning to change unhelpful core beliefs may help you to look at things in a more constructive way and reduce the number of unhelpful thoughts that you experience. It may also help you to set less harsh rules for yourself, which will help you to adopt new ways of behaving that are more consistent with your new, more positive beliefs.

For example, if your core belief was 'I am a failure', your assumption may be along the lines of 'If I don't do well all of the time, then I am not good enough.' As a result of this assumption, it is likely that you would set harsh rules for yourself, and you would rarely be happy as you would be striving so hard to attain perfection. *Perfection is a concept that doesn't fit reality.* You would also probably be very self-critical and be unwilling to try new activities for fear of making mistakes.

However, if you were able to challenge your negative core belief and develop a new one, such as 'I am good enough' your assumption might be something like 'If I put a reasonable amount of effort into all that I do, then I will be successful some of the time.' It is likely that you would set yourself less harsh rules and that you would therefore be more willing to accept mistakes, be pleased about things that you achieve, and be more inclined to take risks and to try new things.

How Do I Identify Assumptions and Core Beliefs about Myself?

There are two methods of doing this, either one of which you might find helpful.

First, try looking back at some of the unhelpful thoughts that you wrote down in your unhelpful thoughts and new thoughts diaries, to see if there are any themes that occur repeatedly. If there are some common themes, they might provide you with some clues. For example, if you notice that a lot of your unhelpful thoughts are related to not managing to do things as well as you would have liked or not achieving your targets, your theme may be to do with being not good enough/a failure/incompetent, etc.

If you are unable to find a particular theme from looking at your unhelpful thoughts, then you may find the second technique more helpful. This is what we call the 'downward arrow' technique.

The Downward Arrow Technique

- First, find an unhelpful thought about yourself in your unhelpful thoughts diary or new thoughts diary, one that was associated with an intense emotion.

- Write down the situation where you had the unhelpful thought, and the thought itself. Then ask yourself: 'What does this say or mean about me?'
- Keep asking the same question of each answer you come up with until you arrive at a core belief about yourself.
- You may only need to ask the above question once or twice to arrive at a core belief; on the other hand, you may need to ask it three or four times.

Here is an example of how a core belief is identified using the downward arrow technique.

Example of an unhelpful core belief about 'me'

Situation	You are called in to see your boss at work
Thought	He doesn't think my work is good enough, I'm bound to get the sack
Question	'What does this say or mean about me?'
Answer	I'm no good at my job
Question	'What does this say or mean about me?'
Answer	I'm no good at anything
Question	'What does this say or mean about me?'
Answer:	I am incompetent – *core belief.*

A blank copy of an 'Identifying Core Beliefs worksheet' setting out this process is provided on page 116 for you to photocopy and fill in.

Sometimes, identifying core beliefs about yourself will be enough to enable you to understand a recurrent problem in your life. However, identifying and challenging unhelpful core beliefs about others too may help you to get things into better perspective. For example, having a core belief that 'everyone is more competent than me' could compound the core belief about you being 'incompetent'. If you can change your belief to 'others are not competent all of the time', this may help you to see things in context and to feel less 'incompetent'.

How Do I Identify Core Beliefs About Other People?

You can find core beliefs connected with other people using the same guidelines given above for identifying core beliefs about yourself. Instead of starting with an unhelpful thought about yourself, find one that is connected with other people. Again, a blank worksheet is provided on page 117.

Example of an unhelpful core belief about other people

Situation	You are at a get-together with old school friends. They are all talking about their 'interesting' lives
Thought	They all lead far more interesting lives than me
Question	'What does this say or mean about other people?'
Answer	They are more interesting than me
Question	'What does this say or mean about other people?'
Answer	They are better than me.
Question	'What does this say or mean about me?'
Answer	Other people are better than me – *core belief*.

It can sometimes be helpful to try to understand where particular thoughts, beliefs, and assumptions have come from and the effects they may have on you. The chart on page 118 gives an example of how a person's core belief may be formed and maintained. A blank version of the chart is given on page 119 in which you may fill in an example of your own, if you wish.

We would suggest that you particularly focus on the lower six boxes of the diagram as you can do some constructive work on these sections. Thinking about background information that may have led to the development of your core belief helps you to understand the origin of your beliefs but spending too long on this (the top box) may make you feel unhappy or distressed, particularly if you have had traumatic or difficult experiences, rather than encouraging you to look forward to how things might be improved.

Worksheet: Identifying core beliefs about me

Situation:

Unhelpful thought:

Question: What does this say or mean about me?

Answer: _____

Question: What does this say or mean about me?

Answer: _____

Question: What does this say or mean about me?

Answer: _____

Question: What does this say or mean about me?

Core belief:

Worksheet: Identifying core beliefs about other people

Situation:

Unhelpful thought:

Question: What does this say or mean about others?

Answer: _____

Question: What does this say or mean about others?

Answer: _____

Question: What does this say or mean about others?

Answer: _____

Question: What does this say or mean about others?

Core belief:

Example of how core beliefs may be formed and maintained

Background information
What experiences contributed to the development and maintenance of the core belief?
Criticism from parents & teachers; lack of praise; clever older sibling; being bullied

Unhelpful core belief
What is my most unhelpful core belief?
I am inadequate

Assumptions
Rules that guide my behavior (usually expressed as 'if . . . then' statements)
If I don't: get a good mark/come top of the class/receive praise for my work
Then: I've failed/I'm not good enough

Strategies that maintain my core belief
Have very high standards; avoid asking for help; work very hard; overprepare

Typical situations in which my rules and beliefs may be activated
(a) Reflecting on a meeting
(b) Preparing for a lecture
(c) Reviewing a piece of own work
(d) Meeting new people

Unhelpful automatic thoughts and (emotions)
that may occur in the above situations and reinforce core belief
(a) I must have looked stupid when I got tongue-tied in the meeting (embarrassed)
(b) What if I can't answer all of the questions? (anxious)
(c) I can see a lot of mistakes in my work (upset)
(d) They'll think that I am really boring (sad)

Behavior in response to thoughts
(a) Try to avoid further meetings
(b) Spend excessive time reading around the subject
(c) Throw my work in the bin and start again
(d) Make excuses and leave early/avoid going out

How core beliefs may be formed and maintained

Background information
What experiences contributed to the development and maintenance of the core belief?

Unhelpful core belief
What is my most unhelpful core belief?

Assumptions
Rules that guide my behavior (usually expressed as 'if . . . then' statements)

Strategies that maintain my core belief

Typical situations in which my rules and beliefs may be activated

Unhelpful automatic thoughts and (emotions)
that may occur in the above situations and reinforce core belief

Behavior in response to thoughts

Contesting Core Beliefs

Unhelpful core beliefs can take a lot longer to change than unhelpful thoughts because we require a lot more convincing that beliefs that we hold to be absolutely true are not 100 per cent true. It may take weeks or months to change core beliefs. Nevertheless, you have already learned how to challenge your unhelpful thoughts, so you will have acquired techniques that will help you to question the accuracy of your core beliefs.

There are two main ways of contesting core beliefs:

- Finding evidence that does not support your belief.
- Conducting your own experiments to test whether in fact your existing thoughts, assumptions, and core beliefs do or do not always fit your experiences.

Finding Evidence That a Core Belief Is Not 100 per cent True

- Try to find a piece of evidence every day to indicate that your belief is not true all of the time. The evidence can be anything at all; the examples in the 'contesting core belief record' boxes on page 121 may give you some ideas.
- Each day, write down your piece of evidence on your own contesting core belief record (a blank record sheet is provided on page 123).
- When you are able to find a piece of evidence most days that refutes your belief is true 100 per cent of the time, then try to find two or three pieces of evidence each day.
- When you have a list of about twenty items, look at them and draw your own conclusions about whether your original core belief accurately describes your whole experience.
- When you no longer feel that your unhelpful core belief accurately describes your situation or how you feel (this might be after a few weeks or months), then turn to page 125 to find out how to identify a new and more helpful core belief.

Contesting core belief record, example 1

Unhelpful core belief: I am not good enough

Evidence or experiences that indicate that my core belief is not 100 per cent true all of the time

1 Made a small Christmas cake and it was sold
2 Spent a long time on the phone to a friend who was in difficulty
3 Overheard mother-in-law saying that the dinner was lovely as usual
4 Invited friends I did not know well for lunch
5 Made cakes while making lunch
6 Friend thanked me for advice given

Contesting core belief record, example 2

Unhelpful core belief: I am not acceptable

Evidence or experiences that indicate that my core belief is not 100 per cent true all of the time

1 Neighbour came in for a chat
2 Was given flowers for organizing play
3 Nephews really pleased to see me when I went to sister's
4 Mike said he enjoyed our chats on the way to work
5 Bill offered to change my lock
6 Complimented on the production of musical

Conducting an Experiment to Test Your Core Belief

You can conduct your own experiments to test out whether your core beliefs do in fact always fit your experiences. For example, if your core belief is that you are 'unlikeable', you might contact friends and suggest going out/invite them for a coffee, and so on, or say hello or smile at ten people.

You could make a prediction of what you think may happen and then draw your own conclusions from the results of your experiment. It is likely that you would have a mixed response; some people may respond positively and some negatively. However, it is likely that the results would suggest that your core belief was not 100 per cent true.

If you have a core belief that 'I am never good enough' which leads you to put 100 per cent effort into everything that you do, try to put slightly less effort in and see what happens. For example, if you spend on average one hour cleaning the kitchen, try spending three-quarters of an hour; again, you could predict what you think may happen. Then see what actually does happen. Has anyone noticed? Is the kitchen really that much different? Did you have more time for relaxation?

An experiment may be something that you perform frequently, for example initiating a conversation every day to see how someone responds (to challenge a belief that you are unlikeable), or something that you do less often, for example doing less preparation for a seminar (to challenge a belief that you are not good enough). As well as being a useful way to challenge unhelpful thoughts, beliefs, and assumptions, experiments like this may also be used to help you strengthen more helpful thoughts, assumptions, and core beliefs.

Record your experiments and conclusions using the behavioral experiment record on page 124.

Contesting core belief record

Unhelpful core belief: _____

Evidence or experiences that indicate that my core belief is not 100 per cent true all of the time

1 _____
2 _____
3 _____
4 _____
5 _____
6 _____
7 _____
8 _____
9 _____
10 _____
11 _____
12 _____
13 _____
14 _____
15 _____
16 _____
17 _____
18 _____
19 _____
20 _____

Conclusion: _____

Behavioral experiment record

Date	Thought/belief to be tested	Experiment	Prediction	Outcome of experiment	What have I learned from this experiment?
	Write down the thought or belief that you want to test out	Write down details of the actual experiment	What do you think will happen?	What actually happened?	

Identifying a New Belief

It is time to move on to identifying a new belief when you feel that your 'unhelpful' core belief no longer truly reflects how you feel about yourself (or others). It may take you a few weeks or months to reach this stage.

On the basis of the conclusions that you drew from contesting your core beliefs and conducting behavioral experiments to disprove those beliefs, we hope that you will have developed more realistic and helpful beliefs about yourself and/or others.

A new core belief may be the *opposite* of the old unhelpful core belief. For example:

Old belief:	I am unlikeable	I am incompetent
New belief:	I am likeable	I am competent

This does *not* mean that you have to be likeable/competent to everyone, or all of the time.

Alternatively, a new core belief may change an *absolute* belief to a *qualified* belief. For example:

Old belief:	Everyone is better than me
New belief:	Not everyone is better than me; I am better than some people at certain things

How Do I Record Evidence That Supports an Alternative Belief?

Just as you recorded evidence to indicate that your old 'unhelpful' core belief was not true all of the time, it is important that you find evidence to support and strengthen your belief in your new core belief. You can do this using the 'New core belief record' on page 126.

- First, write out your new core belief in the space provided.
- Then, over the coming weeks, try to record small events and experiences that occur each day and support your new belief. The things that you write down will be very similar to the

New core belief record

New core belief: _____

Evidence or experiences that support my new belief:

1 _____
2 _____
3 _____
4 _____
5 _____
6 _____
7 _____
8 _____
9 _____
10 _____
11 _____
12 _____
13 _____
14 _____
15 _____
16 _____
17 _____
18 _____
19 _____
20 _____

things that you wrote down on your contesting core beliefs record.

- You may also like to record events and positive experiences from your past that support your new belief. This will help you gradually build up confidence in your new belief.
- You could also perform some behavioral experiments to affirm your new belief.

Points to Bear in Mind about Tackling Core Beliefs

- Reducing your belief in 'unhelpful' core beliefs often takes a long time because they may have developed and been reinforced over a long period. Don't be surprised if it takes a lot of time and patience.
- Go at your own pace; do not rush this section.
- Developing and strengthening your new core beliefs can also take time, as you may initially have difficulty in finding experiences that are consistent with them.
- Persevering with contesting unhelpful core beliefs, then strengthening and reinforcing new core beliefs, will positively influence the way you think, feel, and behave.
- There will be times in your life when you feel greater levels of distress; at these times you can expect to have more unhelpful thoughts, and your unhelpful core belief(s) may return. At these times, review all of your work from both sections of this chapter and repeat any of the worksheets necessary to help you to challenge your unhelpful thinking patterns and strengthen your new beliefs.

If this all feels like hard work, don't despair: it will be worth it in the long run!

9

Overcoming Blocks to Recovery

At times you may feel that although you are doing everything possible to help yourself to get better, you are having some problems in making progress. You may be following your program conscientiously but find that you are taking two steps forward and one step backward. This can be extremely frustrating and can sometimes make you feel like doing things as and when you are able rather than following a consistent pattern of activity and rest as recommended in this manual.

In this situation it may be that you are being obstructed by one or more 'blocks'. These may be things of which you are totally unaware, or which you may sense in the back of your mind. If you can confront and deal with them, you will probably find it easier to make better progress.

This chapter presents a list of common blocks, with a few suggestions on how to tackle each of them, including notes on which parts of this book in particular may help you.

Fear about Increased Activity Making You Worse

It is completely understandable that you would worry about increasing your level of activity when you are already feeling fatigued and possibly experiencing pain or other symptoms. Maybe you have increased some activities in the past and felt worse for doing so. Maybe you have received conflicting views on how you should manage your fatigue. Some people may have suggested that you should rest as much as possible, which might confuse you when you are trying to do more.

However, fear associated with activity can impede progress in overcoming your illness, for the following reasons:

- Worry about doing more can prevent you from taking the risks that are necessary to help you to overcome CFS.
- Temporary increases in pain or fatigue that may occur as a direct result of doing more can be misinterpreted as doing yourself permanent harm, and this can then lead you to reduce the amount that you do rather than continue to attempt a gradual increase.

In order to overcome these difficulties you may find it helpful to reread the following sections of the book:

- Chapter 1 may help you to understand your symptoms better.
- Chapter 7 will tell you how to increase your levels of activity *gradually*. It will also reassure you that a slight increase in symptoms is normal when you change what you do, and that any such increase usually lasts only a short time.
- Chapter 8 may help you to challenge any 'worrying' thoughts you may have about your symptoms.

Recapping these chapters will help you to feel more confident about gradually increasing your levels of activity and accepting a temporary increase in symptoms.

Perfectionism

We have already seen how certain personality traits may be among the many contributory factors in chronic fatigue syndrome (see Figure 2.1, page 25). Having extremely high personal standards and expectations of yourself, and feeling distressed if you are unable to meet them, may also form a block to recovery for a number of reasons. If you have this kind of personality, you may:

- try to complete an activity in one go; e.g. writing an essay or painting a room (this is likely to increase your feelings of exhaustion, which may then lead to your taking excessive rest);
- not be able to relax properly, as you feel you 'should' be doing something 'useful';
- avoid new activities or resume old activities for fear of not doing things well enough;
- find it difficult to finish tasks because of excessive doubts that lead you to check things or do things repeatedly and make it difficult for you to move on to another task; e.g. when writing letters or an essay, or doing housework;
- never feel that you have done anything well enough, which may make you feel dissatisfied;
- have an overly active inner critic, tending to focus on the things that you have not done and ignoring all that you have done.

In order to help with this problem, we suggest that you reread Chapter 8. This chapter will help you to understand how your perfectionism affects your symptoms, behavior, and emotions. It will also help you to challenge your unhelpful thoughts and beliefs, which in turn will have positive effects on what you do and how you feel.

A number of other strategies may also be helpful. You could try to:

- write down three things that you managed to do each day, however small they seemed; e.g. did the washing up, phoned a friend, did five minutes' reading;
- praise yourself for things that you have done, rather than criticize yourself for things that you haven't done;
- include pleasurable and fun activities in your day, rather than focus on things you feel you 'should' be doing.

For more ideas read 'Dare To Be Average', a chapter in *Feeling Good* by David Burns; and Chapter 9, 'Self-Bullying and How to Challenge It', in *Overcoming Depression* by Paul Gilbert, in this series. (For details see Chapter 14, 'Useful Resources').

Receiving Benefits or Income Protection

When you are severely restricted by your illness, there is no doubt that the financial support provided through these schemes, whether by the state or an insurance company, is very important. However, in certain situations it may make it difficult for you to change, for the following reasons.

- You may feel trapped by your benefits or policy if the conditions stipulate that you can work only for a few hours a week, can earn only a certain (small) amount a week, or may not do any work at all. Although you may feel that you have improved and are able to do *some* work, you may not want to endanger your financial support, fearing that if you come off benefit or relinquish your income protection you may then find that you cannot manage your work and face future financial problems.
- You may be having to attend regular medical check-ups or appeals; these can be very stressful and time-consuming, and make it more difficult for you to concentrate on gradually increasing your activity levels.
- You may fear having to go back to a job that you know contributed to your becoming ill in the first place.

If you feel that any of the above apply to your situation, then you may find it helpful to read the information on 'Work, Courses, and Resources' in Chapter 14 (page 184). This will give you some information about benefits, income protection, employment and educational schemes, and voluntary work. If you are receiving benefits, you might find it useful to discover more about what you are entitled to; for example, how much you can earn before your benefits stop. You may also find out about 'back-to-work' schemes in your area.

You may want to consider enrolling on a course or doing some voluntary work to build up your stamina and confidence gradually before going back to paid work. If you are worried about your financial position, it may be worth writing down your expenditure and income, with a view to appraising realistically how much leeway you have.

If you are receiving payments under an income protection policy (IP), a number of strategies may be helpful; for example, thinking about the advantages and disadvantages of being on IP. You may find it useful to do this with the aid of the problem-solving sheets on pages 145–7. You may wish to discuss different ways of returning to work with your employer. They may be more than happy for you to return to work in a graded way, starting with just a few hours. Doing some voluntary work or a course may also be an option. This would help to build up your stamina and confidence about being able to work again. Alternatively, if you feel that you do not want to return to your previous job or are unable to, you may consider discussing different settlement options with your employer; for example a redundancy package.

Other Illness

Having another illness on top of chronic fatigue syndrome can be a considerable obstacle to consistent progress. You may have increased pain or other symptoms in addition to your CFS that make it more difficult to stick to a structured activity program or to sleep. If your mood is depressed, this too can increase feelings of fatigue. If you get a lot of recurrent infections, for example of the chest or urinary tract, you are likely to feel even more unwell and may find it difficult to sleep and do your planned activities.

If your sleep is disturbed, you may like to re-read Chapter 6 on 'Improving Your Sleep'. This offers some useful strategies that may help you. You could also read Chapter 11, on

'Managing Setbacks'. If you have an infection that comes and goes, this chapter will help you cope when your symptoms are more severe.

If you are under the care of another health care professional for treatment of another condition, it may be helpful to tell them that you are trying to overcome your chronic fatigue using the cognitive behavioral strategies described in this book.

Conflicting Advice or Different Kinds of Therapy/Diet

There is a lot of conflicting information about what is helpful in overcoming chronic fatigue syndrome. Although there is evidence to support cognitive behavior therapy, some health professionals may suggest other treatments for which there is no evidence. This can be confusing.

Starting new treatments or diets for your CFS while you are trying to follow the advice given in this book can make it more difficult for you to concentrate fully on your program of planned activity and rest. In order to help you focus on the techniques described here, we suggest that you do not seek opinions from other specialists while following the guidelines in this book, unless you experience new symptoms which appear to be unrelated to your CFS. Also, if you avoid starting other treatments for your CFS while you are working through this book, you will have a better idea about what has influenced your improvement, which will equip you better to deal with any future recurrence of symptoms.

The 'Wrong' Kind of Social Support

This may sound like a contradiction! How could any social support be 'wrong'? However, certain kinds of support can make it more difficult for you to move forward. Occasionally, well-meaning friends or relatives may be concerned that your program of planned activities and rest, and some of what it involves, will make your symptoms worse. They may base this view to some extent on past experience. Of course, they will have your best interests at heart, but may be too close to the problem to see it objectively.

If you find that those close to you have this kind of reservation about the program you want to follow, reassure them that you believe this approach to be the right one, and that, although it takes time, there is evidence that it works. You could also ask them to read the information for partners, relatives, and friends in Chapter 15. You may also consider photocopying the chapter for other people who may not understand what you are trying to do; for example, a tutor or an employer. Once a role for them has been negotiated you may notice any tensions gradually fade as they feel more confident about how they can help you; for example, praising you for what you do manage, accompanying you on planned walks.

If you have great difficulty in telling people what you want or don't want, you might find a book on assertiveness helpful; for suggestions see pages 183–4.

A Lack of Social Support

Just as the wrong kind of social support can be unhelpful, so a lack of social support, forcing you to rely entirely on yourself, can make it difficult for you to make progress. If you live alone and have no family members or close friends nearby, you may find it hard to look after yourself properly in practical matters, for example cooking meals and doing the shopping. It may also be more difficult for you to persevere with your program if you have the odd bad day and there is no one to offer you any support or encouragement.

If this situation applies to you and you are greatly restricted by your illness, then it may be helpful to consider talking to neighbours to see if they could help you occasionally. There may be small things that you can do for them in return. You might ask friends who live a little way away whether they could call in from time to time. You could also find out whether there are any local support groups for people with CFS or other related problems.

Cultural Issues

Some cultures have difficulty in accepting certain kinds of illness, particularly if an obvious physical cause cannot be found. If this applies to you, or to those close to you, it may result in your continuing to have many unnecessary tests rather than concentrating on your CBT program. Just because an organic cause for your fatigue cannot be found, this does not mean the physical symptoms you are experiencing are not real. You may find it helpful to review Chapter 1 for a detailed explanation of symptoms. Relatives and friends may find the information in Chapter 15 helpful.

Continuing 'Stressful' Situations

Stress of any sort can make it more difficult for you to make consistent progress, however hard you try. Stress can increase your levels of fatigue and also make it more difficult for you to 'switch off' at bedtime or when you are supposed to be resting or relaxing.

Potentially stressful situations include the following:

- Life events, whether good, bad, or neutral, such as moving house, getting married, bereavement.
- Financial difficulties that may have occurred as a result of your not being able to work, or doing less work.
- Work issues: you may feel that your employer is not very understanding about your CFS. You may find that you have too much work to do in too little time or have too many deadlines to meet.
- Environment: you may live in an uncomfortable, unpleasant, or chaotic environment where it may be difficult to relax. You may feel that your home is in a mess as you have difficulty keeping it tidy, filing papers, mending, and so on. There may be a lot of noise in your home or nearby, perhaps from other occupants, neighbours, or traffic. Your house may be too hot or too cold. You may not get on with the people with whom you live.

135

- Relationship difficulties, with your partner or other family members.
- Loneliness, maybe because you live alone or because you have lost friends or cannot go out very often because of your fatigue.
- Illness of a family member or other problems within the family.

If any of the above situations apply to you, you might find reading Chapter 10 on 'Overcoming Worry, Stress and Anxiety Related to Chronic Fatigue Syndrome' helpful. The section on problem-solving may help you to think about alternative ways of tackling your situation. You may also want to think about planning a short daily time specifically for thinking about how to address your problems: for more information see the section on a 'Problem-Solving Strategy for Reducing Worries at Night' on pages 65–6. Don't forget to set aside time to relax. Discussing worries with a close friend or relative (if appropriate) may be helpful. Finally, make use of any available resources relevant to your particular problem; for example, financial advisers to discuss financial issues, landlords/environmental health department to discuss problematic living conditions.

Breaking through Comfort Zones

If you have had CFS for a number of years, you may have stopped doing a lot of things that you used to do. Some may be big parts of your life, such as working, socializing, or studying. Others may be quite small things, such as paying bills or phoning people. Whenever any of us stop doing things for some time, we lose confidence in our ability to do them. It may be that a lack of confidence in your ability to do things, or worry about things not going according to plan, is stopping you from resuming your former activities.

Again, if you feel that any of this applies to you, you may find it helpful to read Chapter 10 on 'Overcoming Worry, Stress and Anxiety Related to Chronic Fatigue Syndrome' which describes some strategies that will help you to resume old activities and try new ones. In addition, Chapter 8 on 'Overcoming Unhelpful Thinking Patterns' may offer some useful hints.

Finally, write a list of things that you have not done for a long time and put them in order from easy to difficult. Incorporate one or two items from your list into your program each week.

Overcoming Worry, Stress and Anxiety Related to Chronic Fatigue Syndrome

We have already discussed how having CFS (like any long-term illness) can at times be very stressful. Not only are you trying to cope with your illness, but you may also have other concerns such as financial difficulties or family worries, or be trying to get back to work.

Trying to overcome your fatigue problems can be stressful enough in itself, what with changing your routine, filling in diaries, and maybe having a temporary increase in your symptoms as well!

Over the past few months we hope that you have started working towards a variety of targets in order to improve your lifestyle. This may have involved resuming some previous activities, such as going back to work, doing your own shopping, managing the home finances, travelling on public transport, or meeting up with old friends again. As well as resuming some of your previous activities, you may be considering some new enterprises, such as a course at college, a different type of job, or a new hobby.

Although you may be pleased being in a position to start new activities or resume old ones, you may feel a bit worried. Questions people frequently ask themselves include the following:

- 'Will I be able to do the work?'
- 'How will I cope with meeting new people at college for the first time when I haven't met anyone new for so long?'

- 'How will I cope on the train? I haven't travelled alone for ages.'
- 'How will I get on with my old friends? I haven't seen them for such a long time.'

Asking oneself these questions is perfectly normal, because when we don't practise something regularly we naturally lose confidence in our own ability to do it, and often when we try new things we are naturally apprehensive.

These worries may trigger feelings of anxiety. We have already discussed some of the effects of anxiety in the section of Chapter 1 on 'Autonomic Arousal in Chronic Fatigue Syndrome'. Figures 10.1 and 10.2 provide further illustrations.

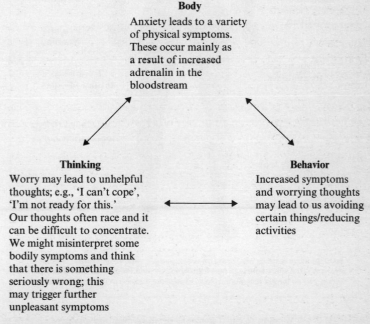

Body
Anxiety leads to a variety of physical symptoms. These occur mainly as a result of increased adrenalin in the bloodstream

Thinking
Worry may lead to unhelpful thoughts; e.g., 'I can't cope', 'I'm not ready for this.' Our thoughts often race and it can be difficult to concentrate. We might misinterpret some bodily symptoms and think that there is something seriously wrong; this may trigger further unpleasant symptoms

Behavior
Increased symptoms and worrying thoughts may lead to us avoiding certain things/reducing activities

Figure 10.1   How anxiety affects us

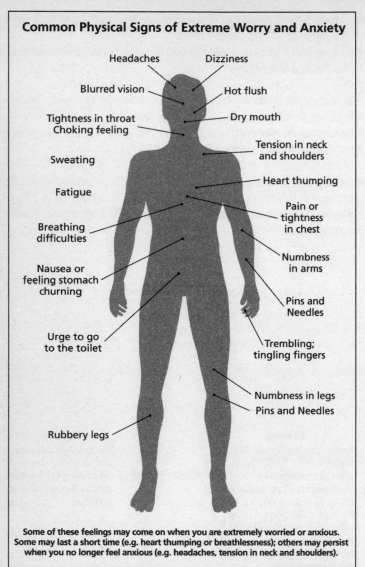

Common Physical Signs of Extreme Worry and Anxiety

Headaches

Dizziness

Blurred vision

Hot flush

Tightness in throat
Choking feeling

Dry mouth

Tension in neck
and shoulders

Sweating

Heart thumping

Fatigue

Pain or
tightness
in chest

Breathing
difficulties

Numbness
in arms

Nausea or
feeling stomach
churning

Pins and
Needles

Urge to go
to the toilet

Trembling;
tingling fingers

Numbness in legs
Pins and Needles

Rubbery legs

Some of these feelings may come on when you are extremely worried or anxious.
Some may last a short time (e.g. heart thumping or breathlessness); others may persist
when you no longer feel anxious (e.g. headaches, tension in neck and shoulders).

Figure 10.2   *Common physical signs of extreme worry and anxiety*

Common Worries Associated with Chronic Fatigue Syndrome

Listed below are some of the worries that people suffering from chronic fatigue syndrome most frequently report:

Resuming previous activities/responsibilities
- going back to work
- managing the home
- driving
- making contact with old friends

Starting a new activity
- a new job
- a course at college/university
- making new friends

The meaning of symptoms
- how to interpret symptoms
- what to do about them
- how to get the activity level 'right'

Giving up benefits/disability allowances
- financial concerns
- loss of disabled parking permit, resulting in not being able to park the car near to shops, etc.

Difficulty in making decisions
- large decisions such as whether to return to the same job or to apply for a new one
- small decisions such as whether going away for a weekend will be counterproductive

Not knowing what to tell prospective employers
- whether to tell prospective employers about their chronic fatigue problems or not

Feeling responsible or blaming oneself for the illness and the effect that it has on others

- if life has changed considerably; e.g. a partner does all the domestic chores as well as working
- if there is a loss of earnings leading to financial difficulties
- if children are not having as much attention as they used to do

How to Deal with Your Worries

In this section we are going to suggest two different ways, both tried and tested, of helping you to overcome your worries. We suggest that before embarking on either of them you spend a while reading through the chapter as this will help you to decide which of the strategies is likely to be most helpful to you.

Whichever strategy you decide to try, the process will take the same four-step form, as outlined below.

Step 1: Write any situations or activities that worry you in the space provided below.

1

2

3

4

5

6

7

Step 2: Look at your list and decide what you would like to tackle first. It may be helpful if you start by tackling the things that cause you the least worry and move on to the more difficult situations as you gain confidence.

Step 3: Decide whether A or B (on the next page) is the best way of helping you to tackle each of your difficulties. (You may decide to use different strategies for different worries.)

A *Problem-solving*
  This is a process that can help you decide what you want and how to go about it.
B *Exposure to situations that cause anxiety*
  This is a process that can help you to face situations that make you feel anxious.

Step 4: Include a regular allocation of time to tackle your difficulties when you write your next activity program.

A: Problem-Solving

Define the Problem

What is your problem? Try to define it as clearly and objectively as possible, and write it down so you can easily follow the steps outlined below to solve it. Defining a problem clearly can take some time, but vague ideas about it may lead you to pursue a solution that is off-track! If your feel stuck identifying a precise problem statement you may find it helpful to have a chat with a friend or partner about it. Other people can be more objective and may be able to help you identify the problem more clearly.

Propose Alternative Solutions

Think of at least three alternative ways of solving the problem. This is important, as the first solution you think of may not be the best one.
  If you have difficulty thinking of any alternative solutions:

• Try to see the problem from someone else's point of view by asking the question, 'If ____ were in my shoes, what would he or she do?'
• Use the point of view of someone that you feel has dealt well with a similar problem, or someone you feel is good at solving problems.
• Try to think how you solved a similar problem in the past.

Evaluate Your Alternative Solutions

Once you have thought of as many alternative solutions as possible, the next step is to evaluate the possible outcome(s) of each one. Do this by writing down what you think the *positive* and *negative* consequence(s) of each of your alternative solutions might be.

Make a Decision

Now that you have considered the possible outcome of each solution, it is time to make a decision on which solution to the problem seems to be the best. Don't forget to consider the practical question: Is it achievable?

Make a Plan and Implement the Solution

What this stage involves will vary according to the type of problem you are trying to solve. It may be that no planning is needed as it just involves saying something to someone; on the other hand, you may need to make a detailed plan of action in several stages.

Evaluate your Plan and Alternative Solution

Once you have tackled your problem by putting into action your chosen 'alternative solution', ask yourself the following questions:

- Did I follow my proposed plan in tackling the problem (if a plan was made)?
- Did the outcome that I expected to occur happen?
- Am I satisfied with the outcome?
- Would I use the same strategy/strategies again?

Solving problems in this way can seem rather long-winded and laborious, but once you have used the problem-solving technique a few times, you may be able to solve the problems in your head without the need to write anything down.

Two examples of the problem-solving technique in use are given, followed by a blank problem-solving sheet for you to photocopy and use.

Problem-solving in action: example (1)

Problem definition
Difficulty coping with inconsiderate lodger.

Alternative solutions (Think of at least three)	*Evaluation of alternative solutions* (What is a possible outcome of each alternative solution?)
1 Put up with it.	1 I need the money from rent. Inactivity is unlikely to help.
2 Ask him to leave and find a new home.	2 Next lodger may be no better. May not find one for a while which would lead to money problems.
3 Discuss problems with him.	3 This will kill or cure problem.

Decision on best solution
3 Discuss problems
with him.

Make a detailed plan
When he returns home from work, say that I would like to speak to him at his convenience.
Discuss the points that I find difficult about him.
Agree that we can review the situation again in six weeks.

Evaluation of plan
Worked well. Agreed to speak in six weeks' time.

Problem-solving in action: example (2)

Problem definition
Worried about how I will cope at college, whether I will be able to keep up with the work.

Alternative solutions (Think of at least three)	*Evaluation of alternative solutions* (What is a possible outcome of each alternative solution?)
1 Speak to tutor about my problems.	1 May help my tutor to understand my difficulties and be sympathetic if I am unable to meet deadlines. But it may make me feel different from others. Do I want that?
2 Put off course for a few months.	2 Although I may feel a little better then, I may not be that much better, and I would still have to face the problem at some time.
3 Ensure a well-balanced program with planned study time and a mixture of activities and relaxation.	3 This will ensure that I work steadily at my course work as well as have time for other activities and relaxation. Be prepared to be more tired initially.

Decision on best solution
3: Ensure a well-balanced program with planned study time and a mixture of other activities and relaxation.

Make a detailed plan
Find out at college how much course work I will be expected to do each week/term.
Review my current activity program and include regular time for studying. Try to study for short times frequently rather than for long periods occasionally.
Ensure that my program includes a mixture of activities with relaxation time.

Evaluation of plan
It will not be immediately clear whether my solution was the best one as it is likely that I will be more tired initially when I start my course (as with any new activity). Review the situation after a couple of weeks and amend my activity program, if necessary.

If after a month, I feel that I am struggling, then it may be helpful to discuss my difficulties with my tutor.

Problem-solving in action

Problem definition

Alternative solutions (Think of at least three)	*Evaluation of alternative solutions* (What is a possible outcome of each alternative solution?)
1	1
2	2
3	3
4	4

Decision on best solution

Make a detailed plan

Evaluation of plan

B: Exposure to Situations that Cause Anxiety

If you have had CFS for a long time, it is probable that you will have got out of the practice of doing certain things. These may be small things, such as taking responsibility for paying the household expenses, or making phone calls; or they may be bigger things, such as driving a car, giving a presentation at work, or having people round for a meal. If you don't practise things regularly it's easy to lose confidence in yourself – and this can happen quite quickly.

We have all been in situations where we have felt anxious initially; for example, on our first day at school or work, getting married, attending interviews. However, after a few minutes of being in an 'anxiety-provoking' situation, we usually start to feel better and are able to concentrate on the matter in hand. This is because anxiety comes down naturally over time. 'Exposure therapy' makes use of this fact and can be a very effective way of overcoming anxiety. It involves repeatedly confronting situations that make you feel anxious until the anxiety subsides.

The following guidelines will help you overcome anxiety in particular situations.

Write a List of All the Situations that Cause You Anxiety

Write them in order from the least difficult to the most difficult, and start with the easiest thing on your list.

Plan Specific Tasks to Do at Regular Times and as Frequently as Possible

Write down the tasks that you choose in your activity program. What these are will obviously depend on the situation that makes you feel anxious.

For example, if you have lost confidence in your ability to socialize and have lost contact with most of your friends, you might decide to start facing this difficulty by phoning a friend and talking for 15 minutes three times a week. Once you feel that you are managing this exposure task with little anxiety, then you can move on to the next step on your list.

Stay in the Situation until Your Anxiety Subsides

Although feeling anxious is uncomfortable, it is not harmful. Do not leave the situation until your anxiety goes down and you feel a little better.

Expect to Feel Anxious

When confronting situations that you have not entered for some time, it is likely that you will feel anxious for a while. Wait and give these feelings time to pass. Remember that these feelings are nothing more than an exaggeration of quite normal bodily reactions to stress.

Keep a Record of Your 'Exposure Tasks'

This will enable you to track your progress of facing 'difficult' situations. Over time you will notice a decrease in the level of your anxiety and be in a position to move on to the more difficult things on your list. Although the exposure record asks you to rate your anxiety level before, during, and after each exposure task, you may want to make a note of your scores on a notepad that you keep with you, and write them down on your record at a convenient time.

An example of a completed exposure task record of someone who felt anxious in social situations, and a blank one for you to photocopy, are given on pages 150–51.

Sample completed exposure task record

Please record your activities and rate how 'anxious' you feel before, during and after each 'exposure' task, using the scale below.

0	1	2	3	4	5	6	7	8
No anxiety/distress		Slight		Moderate		Marked		Severe anxiety/distress

Date	Time Start/finish	Task	Before	During	After	COMMENTS
14.01.05	9.30–10.30	Have 1 friend round for coffee	5	3	0	Went well, after initial anxiety
17.01.05	10.30–11.00	2 friends for coffee	4	2	0	Felt less worried to start with. Enjoyed myself.
20.01.05	12.00–2.00	Meet friend for lunch	6	3	1	Felt flustered, couldn't park and was late. Then felt OK after a while. Need to get a street map!
25.01.05	11.00–12.00	Meet friend for coffee	3	2	0	Challenge my thoughts about being unreliable!
28.01.05	1.30–3.00	Meet friend for lunch again	2	1	0	Went well. Feel I can move on to next step.

Exposure task record

Please record your activities and rate how 'anxious' you feel before, during and after each 'exposure' task, using the scale below.

0	1	2	3	4	5	6	7	8
No anxiety/ distress		Slight		Moderate		Marked		Severe anxiety/distress

Date	Time Start/Finish	Task	Before	During	After	COMMENTS

Points to Bear in Mind When Tackling Worries, Stress, and Anxiety Related to CFS

- You may need to practise the techniques a few times to gain any benefit from them.
- You may need to use more than one of the techniques to overcome a particular worry. For example, if one of your worries is whether or not to do a course, you may need to try problem-solving to make a decision. Once you have made a decision, you may then need to do some exposure tasks if you feel anxious about meeting new people, undertaking course work, etc.
- As a result of trying to tackle your worries you may notice that you have an increased number of unhelpful thoughts. This is very understandable when you are confronting difficult situations. It is therefore important that you challenge any unhelpful thoughts on your new thoughts record. You may find it helpful to reread Chapter 8.
- Make sure that you plan time to tackle your worries and write down your tasks on your activity program. For example, if you have worries about finances and feel that you need to do some problem-solving, then allow half an hour a day for this on your program.

11

Managing Setbacks

There may be times when you have a setback; that is, an increase in symptoms for more than a day or two. Although this may seem a disaster at the time, it can help you to gain a better understanding of your chronic fatigue syndrome and enhance the way that you deal with it in the future. Most people overcome their setbacks quite easily and go on to make further progress. The important thing is not to panic!

A setback may occur when you are working through this book, or after you have finished. If you have a setback, you may feel that you are sliding backwards and that, instead of maintaining your levels of activity, you are returning to old patterns; for example, resting in response to symptoms, sleeping in the day, or overdoing it when you have a bit of energy. You may feel despondent and be uncertain what to do for the best.

It is important to understand that a setback cannot always be avoided, but it can be dealt with quite easily. The key thing is to be able to recognize a setback if it occurs, and to tackle it by taking some positive action.

Common Triggers of Setbacks

Setbacks can occur for no particular reason, but there are times when they are more likely to occur than at others. The situations listed on the next page can increase fatigue and limit the opportunities to continue regular planned activities and relaxation.

153

- Getting an infection or another illness.
- Experiencing any major life event; e.g. moving house, a bereavement, changing jobs, getting married or divorced.
- Stressful conditions; e.g. if you have builders/decorators working at your home, you have deadlines to meet at work or college, or a member of the family is ill.
- Depressed mood.
- Ceasing to use the techniques described in this book and resuming old patterns of behavior.

Any of these situations can increase fatigue and limit the opportunities to continue regular planned activities and relaxation.

How to Tackle Setbacks

Listed below are a variety of strategies to help you tackle your setback and get back on track.

- If you have a temperature or another illness on top of your CFS, it is important that you increase your rest for a day or so until your temperature returns to normal. Do *not* be tempted to rest for longer, or until all of your symptoms subside, as this may prolong your recovery.
- Try to nip your problems in the bud as soon as you realize that you are not managing so well with your program, as it will then take you less time to get back on track again.
- Prioritize your activities; if you do not have time to carry out your program or do not feel able to do so, do not give up, but modify it until you can get back on course again.
- Remember to balance your days as much as possible in terms of a variety of activities and relaxation.
- Lower your expectations of what you can manage, and praise yourself for any achievements.
- Discuss your concerns with a family member or a friend.
- If your symptoms persist for more than a few weeks, then make an appointment to see your GP.

What if I Have a Setback after Finishing Working through the Book?

- Go back to basics. Review all of the information in the book, but initially focus on Chapter 6 ('Improving Your Sleep') and Chapter 7 ('Planning Activity and Rest').
- It may be worth keeping an activity diary and a sleep diary (if sleep is a problem) for a week, to identify your patterns of activity, rest, and sleep.
- Using the information in your activity diary and sleep diary, construct a basic activity program to tackle the problem areas.
- Ensure that you plan manageable chunks of a variety of activities, with regular relaxation/rest periods.
- In order to monitor your progress, you may like to continue to record your activities on an activity diary or on a target achievement record for a few weeks, or until you feel a bit better again.
- If you continue to have problems overcoming a setback after trying these methods, contact your GP.
- Refer to the information above about how to tackle setbacks and also read your own setback plan, as described in Chapter 13 (see page 182).

PART THREE

Making Further Progress

Introduction

We hope that by the time you reach this part of the book you will have found some useful ways of managing your chronic fatigue syndrome and be feeling that you are on your way to recovery.

This part of the book aims to help you to evaluate your progress, identify remaining problem areas, and learn how to consolidate gains and make further progress. To help you in these reflections, we have included an initial chapter setting out three case studies to show how other people have tackled the problems associated with CFS and attempted to overcome them.

We suggest that you start working through this part of the book once you are feeling a little better, are well on your way to achieving some of your targets, and feel that you no longer need to follow such a rigid regime of diary-keeping.

12

Case Studies

This chapter sets out three case studies of people who received cognitive behavioral therapy for their CFS at the chronic fatigue research and treatment unit at King's College Hospital, London (KCH). Their names and some details have been changed to ensure anonymity. We have chosen these three particular cases to reflect the diversity of problems associated with CFS.

Case 1: Alison

Alison was a 43-year-old married woman who lived with her husband and 10-year-old son. Before attending KCH she had had CFS for six years. She dated the onset to a series of chest infections that occurred over a three-month period. Despite her infections, she pushed herself to continue to work as a nursery school teacher as she didn't want to let down the children in her care or other staff members. However, during that Christmas holiday she developed flu and went to bed for two weeks. She found returning to work in the New Year very difficult. Her limbs ached and she felt exhausted all the time. She had frequent sore throats and headaches. Her memory and concentration were poor, and she became distressed that she could not always remember the names of the children or other teachers. She gave up her job after a couple of months as she felt unable to cope any longer.

The next few years were very difficult for her. She spent a lot of time resting in the day, but had difficulty sleeping at night. She tried to 'put on a brave face' and be active when her son returned from school, but found this increasingly difficult. She felt upset and frustrated that she was not able to do simple things like the shopping or heavy housework as they were too exhausting. Her husband became resentful that he was having to work hard in the day and do chores in the evenings and weekends. She began to feel demoralized, fearing that her once active and happy life was slipping away. Her circle of friends gradually reduced as she rarely felt well enough to go out. Over the years she had seen a variety of doctors and had a number of tests, all of which showed nothing abnormal. Rather than feeling comforted by this, she felt upset that while she was feeling so unwell no one could explain why.

When Alison first attended KCH she was in a wheelchair as she was only able to walk for about two minutes at a time without needing to sit down. As with all patients, a detailed history was taken and a diagnosis of CFS was confirmed. We discussed the factors that might have contributed to the onset of her CFS, as well as those that maintained it. We agreed that contributing factors may have included a busy lifestyle, being a working mother as well as having a demanding job, and suffering recurrent infections during which she took no time off. Her fatigue was initially maintained by pushing herself too hard without taking time out to rest. However, when she gave up work she rested for a lot of the time, which contributed to a gradual reduction of fitness as well as sleep problems at night. Understandably, she felt demoralized and frustrated at times. She feared that activity would make her feel worse and therefore restricted her activities further. She had lost confidence, which resulted in her giving up previous responsibilities at home, such as paying expenses and looking after the household, and going out with friends.

Alison's CBT treatment initially focused on establishing a consistent pattern of planned activity and rest and a regular sleep routine. Some longer-term targets that she wanted to work towards were also agreed during her sessions. These included walking twice daily for 20 minutes, cooking a meal every night, attending an evening/day class, and going out with friends once a week.

Alison made excellent progress in the first couple of months. She almost reached her target for walking, had taken over the cooking at home again as well as a few more of the household chores, and had gradually cut down some of her resting time. Her sleep had improved as a result of doing more in the day and developing a good pre-sleep routine. Challenging unhelpful thoughts at the fourth session helped her to address her worrying thoughts about her symptoms.

At Alison's sixth session, she felt that the past two weeks had not gone well and that she had reached a plateau. When this was explored further, it transpired that the work that had been done so far had felt 'comfortable', but the next step involved her thinking about doing a course, which caused her a variety of worries. These included what course to do, whether she would be able to cope with the work, and whether she would be able to make friends with the other course members. Her worries were discussed at some length and she was reassured that it was completely normal to feel anxious about doing something that she had not done for a long time. It was stressed that all of us lose confidence in our own ability to do certain things if we don't practise them regularly. During the discussion, it turned out that Alison had always felt a little anxious with new people, and remembered being shy as a child and having some difficulties with mixing with other children. A variety of ways to help her to overcome this 'block' were discussed. First, the effects of anxiety were discussed, in terms of thoughts, behavior, and physical feelings (symptoms). It seemed that attending a college course was a more difficult target to achieve than she had originally thought. Therefore, steps were agreed to help her work towards going to college later that year. Exposure therapy was discussed as a helpful way to reduce anxiety. A list of 'easy' to 'difficult' things that she would need to be able to do in order to go to college were agreed. She was encouraged to include a few of these things in her activity program over the next few weeks. Examples included phoning two friends every week and organizing quotes for two rooms to be decorated. When she achieved these things, she was encouraged to continue working through her list. She tackled her unhelpful 'anxious' thoughts by generating helpful alternatives. Over the next few weeks she began to feel more confident in her ability to get on with people.

Alison was discharged after 14 sessions and then attended three follow-up sessions over the next year. By session 14, she had managed to increase her walks slightly and was resting for only three hours a day as opposed to between six and eight hours when she first attended the hospital. She was seeing friends more regularly, doing more of the housework and shopping, and had registered for a creative writing course. Her relationship with her husband had improved as he had a better understanding of her CFS and was not having to do all of the chores at home. By the time of her three-month follow-up session, Alison was continuing to make progress. She had started the creative writing course and was really enjoying it. She was able to do more with her son, such as go to the park with him, have his friends round for meals, and help him with his homework. By the six-month follow-up session, Alison had taken over most of the things that she had stopped doing at home. By the one-year follow-up appointment, she had returned to part-time work at the nursery school.

Overall, Alison felt that CBT had improved her understanding of CFS and had equipped her with some useful strategies to tackle the problems associated with it. She decided that she did not want to return to full-time work as she was enjoying having some free time and wanted to do some further courses. Her confidence in her ability to get on with people had greatly improved and she had made some new friendships as well as resuming some old ones.

Case 2: John

John was a 52-year-old teacher who lived with his wife. They had one grown-up son who had left home. John had become ill two years before attending the CFS clinic. He dated the onset of the problem to a particularly stressful time at the school where he was head of department. There had been a lot of recent staff changes, particularly in his department, where a couple of teachers had retired. There was also a lot of work pressure associated with exam preparation for the children. Over a period of a few months, he noticed that he was working later than usual at school and also at weekends. One Monday morning, he woke up feeling exhausted. He got out of bed and put it down to 'another bad night'. He managed to keep going for the next few weeks, but then, after catching a heavy cold, decided to take a few days off. His GP gave him a sick note for the last week of term. The first few weeks of the summer holiday were a blur. He slept for a lot of the time, but did not feel any better for it. His GP carried out some blood tests which were all normal. The thought of returning to the school in September terrified him, as he could hardly focus on reading a book for half an hour, let alone teaching 30-plus children. His GP gave him a sick note for a couple of weeks, and then for a month at a time. After a few months he started to receive sickness payments as he was too unwell to return to his job, although he was promised that his post would be available to him at a later date if he was able to return. Over the next couple of years he remained very fatigued and developed a number of other distressing symptoms. He tried a variety of alternative treatments, which gave some temporary relief of his symptoms but did not lead to a significant improvement. He tried to keep active when he had some energy, but he always seemed to overdo it and pay for it over the next few days. He became very frustrated by his lack of progress despite all his efforts.

When he first attended hospital a diagnosis of CFS was confirmed. He was relieved to have a name for all of his symptoms because, although previous doctors had suggested that he might have CFS, other people, including friends and ex-colleagues, suggested that he was just 'stressed out'. A typical day involved him getting up late morning, as he did not feel that there was anything to get up for earlier, and also because his sleep at night was often disturbed, with long wakeful periods. He would try to do a few chores in the afternoon before his wife returned home from work. Some days he would go for a short walk, and when the weather was fine he would try to do some gardening. However, on one or two days a week he would often just lie on the sofa for most of the day. These 'bad' days often followed the weekend, because he would generally be more active when his wife was at home.

CBT for John initially involved regulating his activity and rest pattern and establishing a better sleep routine. Targets he wanted to work towards during CBT were agreed. They included getting up by 8.30 a.m., reading for half an hour twice a day, walking for half an hour every day, and going out socially once a week. He also was very keen to work again, but did not want to make it a target for the time being.

John made good progress in the early part of his CBT program. He found the planned periods of activity and rest very helpful. It meant that, rather than spending a couple of days resting following the weekend, he was able to be more consistent in the amount that he achieved each day. His sleep pattern gradually improved, which was probably the result of sleeping less in the daytime. He gradually managed to get up earlier in the morning by moving his getting-up time back by 15 minutes each fortnight. He became more consistent with his walks and started to enjoy them. He felt more useful at home as he was cooking meals more frequently and doing chores without his wife having to ask him. Challenging unhelpful thoughts helped him to feel less guilty and less frustrated about his situation. It also helped him to see his old friends again because, rather than thinking that he would seem boring to them, or had nothing to contribute to their conversation, he was able to think that they would probably be pleased to see him again regardless of what he talked about. Their friendships went back a long way, after all, and were unlikely to be affected by what he did or didn't talk about.

At about the ninth session, John was making such excellent progress that it was agreed that it would be a good time to begin to discuss work options. This was quite a difficult issue for him. Although he was very keen to work again and to reduce his sickness payments, he wasn't sure what to do. On the one hand, he wanted to return to teaching: this was what he had always done, and for many years he had greatly enjoyed it. On the other hand, teaching had changed in recent years, and now involved a lot more paperwork and many more exams. He also felt that work had been a major contributing factor to the onset of his problems. It was obvious that unless this dilemma was resolved, it would be difficult for John to make progress. Problem-solving was therefore introduced so that John could consider alternative solutions about working again. As this was a major issue for him, this discussion went on over a number of sessions. John discussed the options with family and friends as well as his headmaster. Between sessions, he began to look for alternative work options so that if he did decide not to return to teaching, he could do something else. John finally decided that he would give up teaching and do something new. This decision was a hard one for him, but he was encouraged by a number of people suggesting that moving to pastures new might be a really positive step. Also, when he went to his old school to meet up with the head, he noted that many of his colleagues had left and the place did not feel the same any more.

Before John began attending KCH, medical retirement had been a possible option for him, but he had always believed that one day he would go back to his job. However, when he reached his decision not to return to teaching again, he activated the medical retirement process, supported by his GP and his therapist. He decided that he would do something completely different and decided to try his hand at gardening. He had increasingly enjoyed working in his own garden and had already helped a relative and a neighbour with theirs.

By the time he was discharged, after 14 sessions, John felt that a heavy weight had been lifted from his shoulders. He was feeling quite optimistic about the future. His symptoms had reduced, although he still needed to structure his day carefully to include planned rests in the morning and afternoon. He did not need to sleep in the day, and his sleep at night was sound and more refreshing. He was managing to get up between 8.30 a.m. and 9.00 a.m. each day. As a step to get back to work, he had started doing a few hours of gardening for one or two interested neighbours and friends. At his three-month follow-up appointment, he had completed a six-week gardening course and had registered for another. He had also increased his gardening work and was planning to do some decorating in the winter months to take its place. Despite his progress, he still continued to need to take his planned rests and noticed that when he didn't, he became more fatigued. By the one-year follow-up session, he had advertised locally to do gardening part-time and had completed another landscape design course. He was in the process of no longer needing sickness payments, which greatly pleased him. Although his new lifestyle would mean a bit of a struggle financially, he and his wife agreed that they could manage. During the follow-up period, he had resumed some of his old friendships, as well as making new ones through the landscape gardening course.

Overall, John felt that CBT had helped him to understand and manage his CFS better. He had found all the strategies helpful. Problem-solving especially had really helped him to weigh up the pros and cons of returning to his old job. Despite feeling sad about his decision not to teach again, he realized that he had given some good years to the profession, and did not rule out the possibility of doing a little private tuition in the future. He felt happier and more confident than he had for some time, and was looking forward to the prospect of being self-employed and building up a small landscape gardening business.

Case 3: Jackie

Jackie was a 32-year-old married woman who worked full-time in a demanding research job for a pharmaceutical company. Before attending KCH she had been ill for about three years. She noticed that she was becoming more fatigued over a period of a few months during the winter. She put it down to the 'horrible' weather and carried on as normal. She and her husband went on a skiing trip to help her to overcome her fatigue, but unfortunately on the second day she got food poisoning and spent most of the week in bed. When she returned home, everything seemed more of an effort. Instead of going out in the evening two or three times a week, she could only go out once. Running and going to the gym, which she had previously done three or four times a week, were put on hold. She was trying to work hard as she had some important deadlines to meet, but this was becoming increasingly difficult as she was finding that her concentration and memory were both poor. Over the next few months, she started to take the odd day off, and this caused problems with her boss as she wasn't meeting her deadlines. He became very critical of her, which greatly upset her as she had always tried to do her best. In an attempt to meet her deadlines she stopped doing pretty much everything outside work except resting and sleeping. Her husband was very worried about her and encouraged her to see the doctor. Following blood tests, which did not indicate a reason for her fatigue, she was referred to a medical practitioner for further tests. Eventually she was referred for CBT.

When she first attended KCH, Jackie was still meant to be working full-time, but was managing to go to work only three or four days a week. She had used up most of her quota of sick leave and had started using up her annual leave days too. When she was not at work, she spent most of the time resting or sleeping on the couch. Her sleep at night was poor, and she lay awake for hours worrying about her situation. She felt very demoralized and felt that for the past few years her life had been put on hold. As well as constant fatigue, she experienced muscle soreness, tender glands, and frequent headaches. She had gained 10 kg (22 lb) in weight in the past two years and felt fat and unattractive. She also felt isolated as she rarely went out and her husband was sometimes away on business trips.

A diagnosis of CFS was confirmed at her first appointment. Factors that might have contributed to the onset of her fatigue and those that maintained it were discussed. It was agreed that a combination of burning the candle at both ends (i.e. working hard, socializing, and exercising excessively) might have played an important part in contributing to her fatigue. The stomach bug that she developed while she was away on holiday was like the straw that broke the camel's back. It was agreed that a combination of a 'boom and bust' approach to activity (i.e. working excessively to meet her deadlines and please her boss and then resting for long periods) were important factors in keeping her CFS going. Other maintaining factors included an erratic sleep pattern and loss of fitness resulting from reduced physical activity. Fewer pleasurable activities, difficulties with her boss, and a poor self-image had made her feel demoralized and low, which had also contributed to increased feelings of fatigue and a lack of desire to see friends.

CBT for Jackie initially involved establishing a more regular pattern of activity and rest and developing a better sleep routine. This involved her taking a 15-minute break in the morning, a 30-minute lunch break, and a 15-minute break in the afternoon. It was agreed that she would go for two ten-minute walks each day. She did this by getting off the bus one stop earlier in the morning and getting on the bus one stop later after work. At weekends, or days when she did not work, she planned to walk to the local stores a couple of times a day. It was agreed that she should sit down and do something relaxing for an hour in the early evening before preparing a meal. To establish a better sleep routine, she was encouraged to try not to sleep during the day and not to go to bed too early, that is, not before 10 p.m. To reduce her worries at night, she was encouraged to set aside a few minutes in the early evening to 'problem-solve' any issues that were likely to bother her at night. If she was not asleep within about 20 minutes of going to bed, she was encouraged to get up so that she would begin to reassociate bed with sleep rather than being awake. A getting-up time of 8.00 a.m. was agreed. Targets that she wanted to work towards were discussed. Although she was keen to resume her previous busy lifestyle, with lots of social and sporting activities, she was advised against this, because her previous extremely busy lifestyle was likely to have been a major contributing factor to her developing CFS. Instead, a compromise was reached and she decided that while she would still like to go out twice a week, one of her outings would be to see a film, which would be less demanding than a sporting activity. She decided that rather than strive for a goal of running or going to the gym again, she would focus on building up her walking and then think about a more energetic goal at a later date. Another goal was to resume a full working week; and her final goal was to be able to go away for a weekend with her husband, or to have people to stay, once a month.

Although Jackie tried very hard to follow the agreed program, she found it very difficult. The main reason for this was feeling guilty about taking breaks at work because of her concerns about what her colleagues or her boss might think. She therefore took breaks only on one or two of the days at work, and continued to feel exhausted when she got home. On the days that she did take her planned breaks, she noticed that she felt better in the evenings, didn't fall asleep on the sofa, and slept better at night. It was therefore discussed at session four how to increase the likelihood of her taking her planned breaks at work. It was first agreed that the therapist would write to Jackie's boss to explain why she needed to take these breaks. Jackie had already tried to talk to her boss, but as he didn't have a very clear understanding of her CFS, this conversation had not gone well. Discussion of the role of unhelpful thoughts affecting how we feel and act was a great help to Jackie. Talking about an example of an unhelpful thought that Jackie was having about work ('My boss will think I am playing truant') helped her to see the thinking errors that she was making. She was then able to come up with some more helpful alternatives.

Over the next few weeks she began to make more progress; she was managing to take breaks at work (the letter to her boss had been helpful), she had stopped sleeping in the day, and she was finding her walks easier. She was a little more active at weekends, although she hadn't yet had friends round or been away. Then, after a month of sustained improvement, she got flu and went to bed for a week. She cancelled a couple of appointments, and when the therapist spoke to her on the phone she was very upset and felt that she had gone back to square one. At Jackie's next appointment, the therapist discussed with her how setbacks can happen and showed her that, rather than seeing them as entirely negative, it was useful to look at them as an opportunity to understand and deal with the illness better. The therapist discussed common triggers such as infections and major life events. Jackie then discussed with the therapist how to tackle any future setbacks; for example, by gradually increasing activities again, pacing herself, not expecting too much of herself.

By the next session, Jackie had almost resumed her pre-flu level of activity and was quite pleased about this. However, it was clear that there were a number of unhelpful thoughts that she had been challenging over the past few weeks that seemed to revolve around a similar theme of not doing well enough. When this was explored further, Jackie said that she had never felt that she was able to do things well enough as this was the message that she had received when growing up. She had always striven to do her best, which at that time meant working very hard at school to get good grades in her exams. When she did not manage to get into Oxford University, her father was disappointed, as he had studied there. Having CFS had compounded her worst fears about not being good enough, and they were further reinforced by her critical boss. Drawing a diagram of how core beliefs may be formed and maintained was a useful first step in helping her to understand the effects of this belief that she had had for many years. Over the coming weeks, she began to challenge this core belief by finding evidence that didn't support it. She also carried out small experiments to test her beliefs, such as not checking her work through more than once (she had used to check everything she did at least five times, fearing a mistake and criticism). Although her progress

170

was slow, she gradually started to believe that she was good enough some of the time. Her progress speeded up when she began to challenge another core belief, that 'others are better than me'. This belief had also stemmed from her early years, for she had had two clever elder brothers; and it had been further reinforced by her being placed in the lower end of a very competitive school.

By the time Jackie was discharged, after 12 sessions, she felt much better. She was working five days a week, and had negotiated an agreement that she could work at home on one of those days. Her sleep was much better, and she had started to see her friends again. However, she had not increased her exercise and therefore had not lost any weight. There had been little overall change between her three- and six-month follow-up appointments, as she had had some work deadlines to meet and pushed herself too hard. This had resulted in her overdoing it again and falling back into old patterns. However, she had managed to get back on track again a couple of weeks before her appointment. Also, between her three- and six-month follow-up appointments she had started to go to the gym again and had lost 3 kg (7 lb). This had greatly pleased her. By her one-year follow-up session, she had been away for a few weekends, which she had enjoyed very much. Her weight had reduced by a further 4 kg (9 lb) and she had treated herself to some new clothes. She had been able to develop new core beliefs of 'I am good enough' and 'I am as good as other people'. However, she continued to need to write things down to strengthen her core beliefs, particularly when she went through a bad patch at work.

Overall, Jackie felt that CBT had changed her life. Understanding the importance of balancing her day between activity and rest and developing a consistent sleep pattern had been helpful. However, she felt that it was identifying her core beliefs, and then understanding the impact that they had on her life, that had really helped her to make progress. Although she still became fatigued from time to time, this happened far less often, and her other symptoms had also decreased markedly.

13

Preparing for the Future

Well done for reaching this part of the book! We hope that by now you will be feeling a little more confident about managing your chronic fatigue problems, be feeling a little better in yourself, and be doing more of what you want to do. However, feeling a bit better can lead to the temptation to let things like planned rests or regular bedtimes slip! This can, as we have already said, lead to a setback which can be rather disappointing.

How Do I Sustain My Improvements and Make Further Ones?

The following suggestions will help you to sustain the improvements that you have made and to make further positive changes to your lifestyle.

- Many activities that were initially part of your activity and rest program are now likely to be part of your daily routine. It is important that they remain so, otherwise there is a risk of sliding backwards.
- If you have targets that you are still working towards, it may be helpful to continue to set yourself an activity program every week or fortnight until they have been achieved. This will help you to remain focused on building upon the improvements that you have already made.

- In order to track your progress, you may find it helpful to continue to keep some sort of record. It is not necessary for you to continue to complete activity diaries or target achievement records unless you find them particularly helpful. We have devised a record that tracks your progress and requires less writing. We have called this a 'Record of progress' and have provided two examples of completed records, followed by a blank one for you to photocopy, on pages 174–6.

How Do I Make Changes to My Lifestyle?

Making changes is an important part of sustaining a lasting improvement. If you don't build on your gains you will find that they evaporate. It is therefore important to set yourself realistic and achievable targets in order to help you to continue to improve your health and lifestyle.

If you have been ill for a long time, not only may you have given up doing many things, such as working and socializing, but other people may have taken over some of your previous responsibilities; for example, shopping, cooking, paying bills, household repairs. If this is the case, readjusting to your previous life can be an alarming prospect. The important thing is to remember to take things gradually and, if necessary, to break them down into manageable steps.

The following guidelines will help to reduce your fatigue and increase your overall energy levels as you embark on these changes.

- Make sure that your lifestyle is balanced between a mixture of different kinds of activity and relaxation.
- Include an hour for yourself each day to do exactly what you *want* to do.
- Ensure that you have regular short breaks when you are working/studying/looking after children, etc.
- Try to ensure that you maintain a regular sleep pattern, by going to bed and getting up at a similar time each day. The

Record of progress, example 1

Week beginning	Program (List activities that I plan for the week)	Comments (How did I get on with my program?)	Plan (What can I do differently next week/fortnight?)
30 June 2004	1 Get up and get dressed by 9 a.m.	Did very well with getting up and going to bed on time	Get up at 8.45 a.m. daily
	2 Have 3 × 1-hour rests	Rested a bit longer than 1 hour each time	Set an alarm clock to make sure that I get up from my rest on time
	3 Go for 3 × 15-minute walks	Didn't manage 3 walks each day	Try to do the 3 walks at regular times; e.g. 10 a.m., 2 p.m. and 6 p.m.
	4 Read 2 × ½ hour daily	Managed planned reading	Increase the reading to 40 minutes × 2 daily
	5 Meet a friend for lunch for 1 hour weekly	Met friend weekly	Meet a friend twice weekly
	6 Go to bed by 11 p.m.		

Record of progress, example 2

Week beginning	Program (List activities that I plan for the week)	Comments (How did I get on with my program?)	Plan (What can I do differently next week/fortnight?)
12 May 2004	1 Try to get back into the routine of going to the gym again on a regular basis. Go to the gym × 3 for ½ hour each week	Managed to go to gym 3 times during the first week and twice in the second week	Did pretty well with my gym attendance. I will try to keep it up during the next fortnight
	2 Go out with friends to celebrate birthday, be home by midnight to avoid too much fatigue following day	Had a good night out, but didn't manage to get home until really late. Felt really awful the next day and therefore didn't go to the gym	Try harder to get home by midnight when I go out to a concert this week, so that I don't miss out on other enjoyable things the day after
	3 Hunt for new flat	Found this really exhausting, but managed to find a new flat	Try to ensure that I have some planned relaxation time of at least 1 hour a day as I am conscious that this is slipping

Record of progress

Week beginning	Program (List activities that I plan for the week)	Comments (How did I get on with my program?)	Plan (What can I do differently next week/fortnight?)

optimal amount of sleep differs from person to person; eight hours a night is about average.

- Aim to do at least 30 minutes' exercise twice a week.
- Prioritize your activities if you find yourself doing too much.

Evaluating Progress

It can be helpful to spend some time thinking about what you have learned from this book and what you need to do in order to make further progress. We therefore suggest that you put half an hour aside at a convenient time to complete the 'Evaluation of progress' form on page 178.

Working towards Current or New Targets

As we have already mentioned, in order to make further progress it is important that you continue to work towards planned targets or devise some new ones. We have therefore included three forms called 'Targets for the next three months'. You can use these forms to write down your targets at three-monthly intervals and to make a plan of how you will work towards them. These forms can be found on pages 179–81.

Managing Setbacks

You will have already read about how to manage a setback in Chapter 11. In order to try to prevent setbacks, or minimize them if they occur, it is helpful to think about your own warning signs of setbacks and strategies that you could implement to deal with them. We have therefore devised a 'Preventing setbacks' form for you to complete; this can be found on page 182.

Evaluation of progress

Please complete the following sections in as much detail as possible.

1(a) What have I learned about CFS?

1(b) What factors may have preceded my CFS?
(e.g. constantly being busy, recurrent infections, aiming for perfection)

1(c) What factors may have contributed to my CFS problem continuing?
(e.g. an erratic sleep pattern, long periods of activity followed by long rests)

2 What strategies have I found helpful while working through this book?
(e.g. having regular breaks, going to bed at a set time, challenging unhelpful thoughts)

3 What areas do I still need to work on?
(e.g. targets I have not yet achieved, resting at regular times, work on core beliefs)

Now please turn to the next page to think about what you would like to work towards in the next three months.

Targets for the next three months

Please write down targets that you plan to work towards during the next three months.

Write a detailed plan of how you aim to work towards each of your targets.

Evaluate your progress at the end of three months and then turn to the next page to plan your targets for the next three months.

Targets for the next three months

Please write down targets that you plan to work towards during the next three months.

Write a detailed plan of how you aim to work towards each of your targets.

Evaluate your progress at the end of three months and then turn to the next page to plan your targets for the next three months.

Targets for the next three months

Please write down targets that you plan to work towards during the next three months.

Write a detailed plan of how you aim to work towards each of your targets.

Preventing setbacks

Review the information in Chapter 11 on 'Managing Setbacks' to help you to complete this sheet.

Can I identify any warning signs that make my CFS worse?
(e.g. when I am very busy/get a cold)

What steps do I need to take if I find myself getting into difficulties?
(e.g. ensure that I take planned breaks, do not stay in bed all day)

14

Useful Resources

In this chapter we provide details of a number of resources that we hope will help you to make further progress. These include useful books, contacts to help in finding work and educational opportunities, information on benefits and where to get advice, and suggestions on how to find specialist help and therapy. For information and professional help in other countries, please see the Appendix.

Further Reading

Many of the books listed below give very good practical advice in overcoming a number of problems that we have not been able to include in much detail.

Martin M. Antony and Richard P. Swinson, *When Perfect Isn't Good Enough: Strategies for Coping with Perfectionism* (New Harbinger Publications, 1998)

Sharon A. Bower and Gordon H. Bower, *Asserting Yourself: A Practical Guide for Positive Change*, 2nd edn (Perseus Books, 1991)

David D. Burns, *Feeling Good* (Avon Books, 1999)

Anne Dickinson, *A Woman In Your Own Right* (Quartet Books, 1982)

Melanie Fennell, *Overcoming Low Self-Esteem: A Self-Help Guide Using Cognitive Behavioral Techniques* (Robinson, 1999)

Paul Gilbert, *Overcoming Depression: A Self-Help Guide Using Cognitive Behavioral Techniques* (Robinson, 2000)

Dennis Greenberger and Christine Padesky, *Mind over Mood* (Guilford Press, 1998)

Helen Kennerley, *Overcoming Anxiety: A Self-Help Guide Using Cognitive Behavioral Techniques* (Robinson, 1997)

Work, Courses, and Resources in the UK

If you are considering returning to work, doing a course, or finding a new job, it can be difficult to know where to start. You may not know what opportunities are available to you. The following details aim to give you some leads to follow.

The Disability Discrimination Act

Many people with CFS, or in recovery from it, are worried about how it may affect either their employment prospects or their current employment. People thinking about future employment are often worried that their illness record or diagnosis will be held against them. People in employment are often concerned that they will be dismissed for taking time off sick, or for being unable to work the amount of hours they used to, or for being unable to perform their previous duties. In fact in the UK most of these concerns are addressed by the Disability Discrimination Act of 1996 (the US equivalent is the Americans with Disabilities Act of 1990).

Who does it cover?
This act defines disability as: 'a physical or mental impairment which has a substantial and long-term adverse effect on [the person's] ability to carry out normal day-to-day activities'. The definition is broad, and covers most cases of CFS. 'Long-term' is defined as either having existed for 12 months or being likely to exist for 12 months after onset. The act also covers those who are in recovery from disability, even if they do not currently fulfil the diagnostic criteria.

What does it do?

The act is a set of guidelines which attempts to protect the recruitment and employment rights of disabled individuals. It also has clauses concerning service providers' obligations to disabled users. We will not describe these latter clauses here. A useful summary of the act is available on http://www.disability.gov.uk/dda/ (see http://www.dol.gov/odep/pubs/foct/ada92fs.htm for the US version). The employment laws apply only to places where 15 or more people are employed.

Recruitment rights are protected in that it is no longer legitimate to discriminate against a job applicant because of their disability history, without justification. Disclosure of a CFS diagnosis and/or related sick time is not then, in general, a legitimate basis for refusing employment, unless the potential employer, after the appropriate advice, considers that the job description is not compatible with the current degree of disability.

If you are already employed and become disabled, it is the responsibility of your employer to make all reasonable attempts to adjust conditions of employment to accommodate your altered ability. Adjustment of employment conditions could include deployment elsewhere within the organization, alterations to an existing role, or changes in working conditions, such as hours worked. Your employer is required to make any such 'reasonable' adjustments and may not refuse to do so 'without justification'.

The terms of the act are not precise and are open to interpretation, for example of what constitutes 'reasonable' and 'justified'.

Information for People Who Are Receiving Benefits

If you have been ill for some time you may be receiving welfare benefits. Understandably, you may have concerns about how your income will be affected if you return to work. You may feel that you are ready for some part-time work, but are unsure about the financial implications.

The following paragraphs summarize the most common benefits claimed by people with chronic fatigue syndrome.

Incapacity benefit (ICB) can be claimed in the UK if:

- statutory sick pay (SSP) has ended or you cannot claim SSP;
- you have paid national insurance (NI) contributions;
- you have been incapable of work because of sickness or disability for at least four days in a row, including weekends and public holidays.

Income support (IS) can be claimed in the UK by people aged between 16 and 59 who:

- are on a low income;
- are not working, or work less than 16 hours a week on average.

Severe disablement allowance (SDA) has not been available to new claimants since April 2001. However, existing claimants can continue to receive it. A person who is incapable of work and who would previously have claimed severe disablement allowance may be able to claim incapacity benefit.

New Work Rules for People on Incapacity Benefit

If you are receiving UK benefits you may be aware that there are rules that determine how much work you can do without your benefits being affected. Below is some information about work rules that were introduced in 2002.

Any person in the UK receiving a benefit on the basis of incapacity (e.g. incapacity benefit, severe disablement allowance, national insurance credits, income support, housing benefit, or council tax benefit) may do paid work for up to 16 hours a week and earn no more than £72 a week for 26 weeks.

In addition to this, a person may be able to do one of the following:

- extend the above for a further 26 weeks if they are working with a job broker, disability employment adviser, or personal

adviser who agrees that an extension is likely to improve their capacity to move into full-time work (i.e. 16 hours or more a week);
- work and earn no more than £20 a week, at any time, without a time limit;
- do supported 'permitted work' and earn no more than £67.50 a week without time limit.

Under the new 'permitted work' rules, the definition of 'supported permitted work' is work that is supervised by someone who is employed by a public/local authority or a voluntary organization, and whose job it is to arrange work for disabled people. This work could be done in the community or in a sheltered workshop. It also includes work done as part of a hospital treatment program.

An eligible person in the UK undertaking work under the permitted work rules will not need their doctor's approval to do so, but they should tell the office that pays their benefit before starting work. As long as the permitted work rules are observed, their earnings will not affect their incapacity benefit and/or severe disablement allowance. However, income support, housing benefit, or council tax benefit could be reduced. It would therefore be advisable to seek advice from the office that pays your benefit before taking a job, so that you are fully informed of your position before starting work.

When permitted work is available, you must apply to the benefits agency to get a permitted work form (PW1).

Income Protection (IP)

IP is a UK insurance scheme whereby you are paid an amount equivalent to part of your salary while you are unable to work. Usually, the policy is held between the employer and the insurance company. Many insurance companies are willing to negotiate a gradual return to work with part payment until full-time work is achieved. Some insurers are willing to pay for rehabilitation and cognitive behavior therapy as a way of helping people to return to work. Some employers will offer redundancy packages on health grounds.

Income protection policies are also available for the self-employed; under these, the insurance company makes regular payments (specified in the policy) if you are unable to pursue your usual work after an initial period of typically one or three months.

Employment and Educational Schemes

Below is a list of UK organizations that you could contact for information and advice on returning to work, finding new work (voluntary or paid), or doing a training or educational course:

WorkCare

WorkCare is a government-funded research initiative that is designed to test innovative rehabilitation and return-to-work services for people who have been off sick. This pilot scheme will provide a boost to the existing healthcare/occupational health and safety services. All services provided by WorkCare are fully funded by the Department for Works and Pensions (DWP) and are therefore completely free of charge. WorkCare is operating pilot schemes in a number of regions including Birmingham, West Kent/South London, Glasgow, Sheffield, Tyneside and Teesside.

You may be eligible if you have been absent from work for between six weeks and six months because of ill health and have a job to return to, but feel unable to in the foreseeable future.

For further information call 0800 052 1659 or visit the website at http://www.workcare.co.uk.

Jobcentre Plus

Jobcentre Plus is a new business within the Department of Work and Pensions. In April 2002 it replaced the employment service (which previously ran jobcentres) and parts of the benefits agency which provided services to people of working age through social security offices. It offers help in both finding work and claiming benefits under one roof.

You can get details of the areas covered by Jobcentre Plus offices from your local Jobcentre Plus, other jobcentres, or social security offices.

For further information visit the website at http://www. jobcentreplus. gov.uk.

New Deal

New Deal is a scheme that gives people claiming benefits the help and support they need to look for work, including training and job preparation. New Deal is part of the Department for Work and Pensions (DWP). Their website, which is listed below, provides information about a number of schemes as well as those listed.

New Deal for Disabled People

New Deal for disabled people aims to give everyone on health-related disability benefits the chance to find rewarding work. Job brokers are available to give you genuine support, tailored to your individual needs. The work will not affect your benefits.

For further information call the NDDP helpline on 0800 137 177 or visit the website at http://www.newdeal.gov.uk/nddp.

New Deal 50 Plus

New Deal for 50 Plus is a valuable package that aims to help people aged fifty or over to find work. You can join the program if you are aged fifty or over and have been receiving one or more of the following benefits for at least six months:

- income support
- job seeker's allowance
- incapacity benefit
- severe disablement allowance
- pension credit

189

You may also be eligible to join New Deal 50 Plus if you have been receiving national insurance credits, invalid care allowance, or bereavement allowance. The program is also available to you if your partner has been receiving an increase in benefits for you for at least six months.

If you join the program, you will get your own personal adviser who will be your main point of contact and support throughout the program.

For further information call 0845 606 2626 or visit their website at http://www.newdeal.gov.uk.

NB: Contact the benefits agency or local jobcentre to find out how it may affect any existing benefits that you are receiving.

Linkline

Linkline is a free telephone helpline service for adults. It provides information and advice on training, learning and work. Linkline can help with the following:

- information on local education courses;
- where and how to get the money you need;
- how to get the right training for a new job;
- where to go to get your CV up to scratch;
- interview skills;
- information on training locally;
- job searching.

For further information call 0800 0641 481.

Learndirect courses and centres

Learndirect offers a variety of courses to do either at home, if you have Internet access, or at one of the many centres in the UK. They can take from 15 minutes to a few hours to complete, but because they are broken down into small chunks, you can work at your own pace.

There are over 750 courses to do in four key areas:

- using information technology (IT);
- information technology (IT) professional;

- skills for life;
- business management.

For further information phone 0800 100 900 or visit the website at http://www.learndirect.co.uk.

Voluntary Work

There are a variety of organizations that may be contacted with a view to finding out about doing voluntary work.

Timebank
Timebank is a national volunteering campaign that:

- offers a number of ways to get involved in your local community;
- runs a number of targeted volunteer initiatives; e.g. in sport, the environment and the arts.

For further information telephone 0845 456 1668 or visit the website at http://www.timebank.org.uk.

UK Volunteering Forum
The UK Volunteering Forum brings together the four national volunteering development agencies in the UK, and offers a range of resources for potential volunteers, volunteer managers, and anyone seeking up-to-date information on volunteering. For further information visit the website at http://www.ukvf.org.

NCVO
The National Council for Voluntary Organizations (NCVO) is the umbrella body for the voluntary sector in England. You can contact the organization by telephoning their help desk on 0800 2798 798 or by visiting their website at http://www.ncvo-vol.org.uk.

Citizens Advice Bureau (CAB)
The Citizens Advice Bureau (CAB) is an organization that gives free, confidential, impartial, and independent advice on a wide range of subjects including employment, benefits, housing, and debt.

For further information contact your nearest CAB by telephoning or dropping in during working hours Monday to Friday. The CAB also has several websites; e.g. http://www.citizensadvice.co.uk.

Website for Information on CFS

The Chronic Fatigue Research and Treatment Unit based at King's College Hospital, London, has a website offering further information about CFS: http://www.kcl.ac.uk/cfs.

Referral to a Specialist

If you have found that the book has helped you, but feel that you would like to be seen by a specialist in CFS, ask your doctor if there is a specialist centre in your area and if you can be referred to it.

Finding a Therapist

If, after working through this book, you would like to have some sessions of cognitive behavior therapy with a therapist, you can ask your doctor to refer you to a qualified therapist in your area who specializes in working with people with CFS. Alternatively you can contact the British Association for Behavioral and Cognitive Psychotherapists (BABCP), which holds a list of accredited therapists who work both privately and in the NHS. You can contact it on the website http://www.babcp.org.uk.

Please note that the information in this chapter was correct and up to date in January 2005.

PART FOUR

How Others Can Help

Introduction

This part of the book has some brief information for people who are close to you. It talks about what chronic fatigue is, how it can affect you, and how they can help.

15

Some Guidelines for Partners, Relatives and Friends

It can be extremely helpful to people suffering from chronic fatigue syndrome (CFS) to have someone near them who understands a little about their problems and the way in which they are trying to tackle them.

The purpose of this chapter is to give you:

• some basic facts about chronic fatigue syndrome;
• guidance on how you can help them to get the best out of this book.

Facts about Chronic Fatigue Syndrome

What is Chronic Fatigue Syndrome?

Chronic fatigue syndrome (CFS), also known as post-viral fatigue syndrome or myalgic encephalitis (ME), is a condition which affects people in different ways. The main symptom is persistent fatigue, which can be severe and disabling, leading to a restricted lifestyle. Other associated problems may include painful muscles and/or joints, sore throats, headaches, dizziness, poor concentration, and memory loss. Problems with sleep are common; for example, sleeping more during the day, having difficulty in going to sleep at night, and waking frequently. Sleep is seldom refreshing.

Fatigue and other symptoms will differ greatly among individuals. As a result of their symptoms, people with CFS may be greatly restricted in their lives. For some, symptoms can be so severe that they remain in bed or rarely leave their home. Others are able to carry out activities for some of the time, for example go to work, look after the home, or do a course of study, but become so exhausted at other times that they are unable to do anything else.

What Causes CFS?

There has been a lot of speculation about different causes of CFS, but it is unlikely that a single cause will ever be identified. However, the following factors seem to be associated with the onset of the illness in many cases:

- an initial illness or a series of infections;
- leading a busy or stressful lifestyle, whether at work or at home;
- stressful life events such as bereavement, moving house, changing jobs, getting married, ending a long-term relationship: all these may lead to increased vulnerability to infections and/or fatigue;
- having high personal expectations and driving to do things 'perfectly': this can be frustrating, causing despondency and fatigue.

What Keeps CFS Going?

People often ask why the CFS keeps on going, months or may be years after the person first became ill. Some of the reasons are listed below.

- Resuming normal activities too soon after an initial infection may sometimes delay recovery.
- Resting too much once an initial infection has subsided can cause its own set of problems. The body becomes out of

condition quite quickly: the muscles, immune system and nervous system are particularly adversely affected. The problems which may ensue include muscle weakness, being more prone to illness, and feeling sluggish, with poor memory and poor concentration.

- Alternating overvigorous exercise with resting for long periods can inadvertently make the problem worse in the longer term, as the body does not get used to a consistent pattern of activity and rest.
- An irregular bedtime or getting-up time, or resting too much in the day, may contribute to disturbed and unrefreshing sleep at night. Not sleeping well at night is likely to increase feelings of fatigue and other symptoms.
- Worries about activity making the illness worse may lead people to stop or reduce certain activities. This restriction of lifestyle in turn can cause them to feel frustrated and demoralized.
- Receiving advice from a variety of sources can lead to confusion and uncertainty about what to do for the best.
- The debilitating effects of CFS can lead to other problems; e.g. financial difficulties, reduced social contacts, or changing roles within the family. These difficulties can understandably trigger feelings such as frustration and helplessness. These feelings, which are a natural human response to stress, can then lead to low mood for some people and depression for others. Low mood itself can lead to a variety of problems including tiredness, which can further reduce the desire to be active.

How Can You Help?

If you are close to someone with CFS who is using this book, your understanding and support can be extremely helpful in assisting them to get better. This book describes a variety of techniques based on cognitive behavior therapy (CBT). This is a pragmatic approach that is helpful to some people with CFS.

The following are some ways in which you may be able to help your partner, relative, or friend.

- Discuss with the person their views on how they best feel that you can help them. It may be that they want you to be significantly involved; e.g. by accompanying them on planned walks, phoning them to make sure they are out of bed, or discussing their progress on a daily basis. On the other hand, they may want to get on with their program by themselves, but want just a little bit of support and encouragement from you.
- Take time to read the information in this chapter so that you understand a little more about CFS and what they are trying to do to overcome it.
- Give praise for any achievements that the person makes, as this is likely to help them to recognize that they are improving. Achievements may be very small; for example, getting up 15 minutes earlier each day, walking for five minutes twice daily, not sleeping during the day, reading the paper for ten minutes a day. All achievements, however small, are signs of improvement.
- Encourage all efforts that the person is making in relation to their program, whether it is doing a particular homework activity, filling in their activity diaries, or reading information in this book. The techniques described in this book are time-consuming and require a lot of effort, so the more support anyone gets for using them the better. Remind them that they can overcome their illness by persevering and that small step-by-step achievements are the key to success.
- When your partner/relative/friend starts to tackle their unhelpful thoughts, they will initially be trying to identify thoughts that may be hampering their progress, such as 'I will never get better' or 'I should be able to do more'. Once the person is able to identify these unhelpful thoughts, they will learn to challenge them and try to think of more 'helpful' or 'positive' alternative thoughts. You may be asked to point out when they say something 'negative' or 'unhelpful'.

Challenging unhelpful thoughts can be difficult as it is not always easy to see a helpful alternative. This particularly applies when someone is feeling poorly, upset, or a bit low. If your partner/relative/friend is struggling, especially if progress is slow, you may be able to help by pointing out some helpful alternatives; e.g. what they have achieved so far.

Please also consider the following points:

- When starting to work through this book, the person may notice an increase in their symptoms. This is usually temporary and occurs as a result of changing their patterns of activity and rest. Encouragement and support at this time are particularly necessary as they may feel like reducing their activities in response to an increase in symptoms. It is important to stress that any increase in symptoms is both normal and temporary, a side effect that occurs because they are changing what they are doing. Encourage them to persevere with the techniques as people usually find that their symptoms gradually decrease and they are able to do the activities with less discomfort and then increase what they are doing.
- Sometimes people want to do too much – usually on 'good' days when they are feeling better. It is important at these times to encourage them to stick to their program, as doing too much and not taking planned rests can lead to an unacceptable level of increased symptoms, delay progress, and lead to a setback.
- If the person wants you to be actively involved in their program, it may be helpful for you both to set aside a regular time each week in which to discuss how they are getting on. This will give you the opportunity to reinforce their achievements, give encouragement when they are having difficulties, and discuss any worries that you have in relation to their program. It is important that you approach any concerns about their program, whether you think they are doing too much or too little, in a non-judgmental manner.

- Setbacks can occur at any time. They are a 'blip' in the recovery phase and certainly do not mean that the strategies described in this book are not helpful. Setbacks are more likely to occur in certain situations; for example, if the person has another illness, moves house, has a bereavement or other distressing experience, or has a number of deadlines to meet. These stressful situations may give rise to increased symptoms and an inability to maintain their program. At these times, it is important to remind the person that setbacks are only temporary. Encourage them to read the appropriate sections of this book in order to get back on track again. Setbacks should be viewed as challenges to be overcome and not as disasters. If a setback occurs after the person has finished working through the book, then encourage them to devise a small activity and rest program for a few weeks, or until they feel they are managing better.
- We hope that, after working through this book, people will be able to do more and need less rest. It is important to encourage them to continue with a balance between different kinds of activities and rest. Breaking this routine, or stopping certain activities, or resting at irregular times may lead to a risk of sliding back. As long as a good balance of activity and rest is maintained, then recovery will be sustained. They may gradually make quite substantial changes to their lives; e.g. returning to work, starting college, or taking over household responsibilities. Although these are all signs of good progress, making these changes can be quite frightening, particularly if the person has been ill for some time. Your support and understanding will almost certainly be appreciated.

Seeking Professional Help Outside the UK

Association for Advancement of Behavior Therapy
305 7th Avenue
16th Floor
New York
NY 10001-6008
USA
Tel.: 212 647 1890
Fax: 212 647 1865
Website: http://www.aabt.org

The Australian Association for Cognitive and Behavior
    Therapy
E-mail: S.Egan@exchange.curtin.edu.au
Website: http://www.aacbt.org/

The European Association for Behavioral and Cognitive
    Therapies has a list of member associations.
E-mail: eabct@vgct.nl
Website: http://www.eabct.com

Index

Order further books in the *Overcoming* series

No. of copies	Title	Price	Total
	Anger and Irritability	£9.99	
	Anorexia Nervosa	£7.99	
	Anxiety	£7.99	
	Bulimia Nervosa and Binge-Eating	£7.99	
	Childhood Trauma	£7.99	
	Compulsive Gambling	£9.99	
	Depression	£7.99	
	Low Self-Esteem	£9.99	
	Mood Swings	£7.99	
	Obsessive-Compulsive Disorder	£9.99	
	Panic	£9.99	
	Relationship Problems	£9.99	
	Sexual Problems	£9.99	
	Social Anxiety and Shyness	£7.99	
	Traumatic Stress	£7.99	
	Weight Problems	£9.99	
	Your Smoking Habit	£9.99	
	P&P & Insurance		£2.50
	Grand Total		£

Name: _____

Address: _____

_____ Postcode: _____

Daytime Tel. No.: _____

E-mail: _____

Three ways to pay:
1. **For express service telephone the TBS order line on 01206 255 800 and quote 'CRBK2'. Order lines are open Monday–Friday 8:30a.m. – 5:30p.m.**
2. I enclose a cheque made payable to **TBS Ltd** for £_____
3. Please charge my ❑ Visa ❑ Mastercard ❑ Amex ❑ Switch (switch issue no. ....) £_____

   Card number: _____

   Expiry date: _____ Signature _____

   (your signature is essential when paying by credit card)

Is/ are the book(s) intended for personal use ❑ or professional use ❑?

Please return forms (*no stamp required*) to, Constable & Robinson Ltd, FREEPOST NAT6619, 3 The Lanchesters, 162 Fulham Palace Road, London W6 9BR. All books subject to availability.

Enquiries to readers@constablerobinson.com
www.constablerobinson.com

Constable & Robinson Ltd (directly or via its agents) may mail or phone you about promotions or products. Tick box if you do not want these from us ❑ or our subsidiaries ❑.